HORMONE RESET DIET

How to Learn the Basic 7 Hormone Diet Strategies with Results in Just 21 Days of Weight Loss and Metabolism Establishment

Alexander Phenix

The content within this book has been derived from various sources. Please consult a licensed professional before attempting any techniques outlined in this book.

By reading this document, the reader agrees that under no circumstances is the author responsible for any losses, direct or indirect, that are incurred as a result of the use of the information contained within this document, including, but not limited to, errors, omissions, or inaccuracies.

Table of Contents

Introduction

When was the last time you looked in the mirror, and we're not okay with the way you look but feel amazing in your own skin, full of energy, and proud of how well your life has turned out?

Let's face it; weight issues are not just vanity problems related to a number on the scale. How you look in the mirror, and the size of clothes you wear is only one tiny aspect of how your entire life functions.

Your weight might be the easiest issue to blame for all your problems, but there's a lot more going on inside your body that is causing the weight gain and retention, not to mention the difficulty sleeping, mood swings, energy slumps, and depressing lack of a sex drive.

The bad news is that exercising more and eating less is not going to solve your problem. That really hard "easy button" that has been the mantra of fitness professionals and conventional doctors for years is obviously not working.

The good news is that balancing your hormones through an easy to follow and sustain nutrition program can truly get to the root of your problems and heal them from the inside out.

By understanding how hormones work inside of your body, you can reestablish the homeostasis, or balance, that your body needs to keep you running at maximum efficiency day in and day out.

If you can reset your hormones to their factory perfect settings, you can finally lose the stubborn weight that has been following you around for far too long. More importantly, you'll also increase your energy, improve your sleep quality, support your brain function and mental health, and reduce your stress levels dramatically.

Essentially, by resetting your hormones so that they're optimally balanced, the rest of your life will start to feel more balanced as well.

What is a Hormonal Reset

It can be surprisingly simple to reset your hormones if you know what you're doing or, in this case, have a guide to follow. Your body wants to be in balance, and it will naturally do everything in its power to return to homeostasis. All you have to do is stop getting in its way.

Unfortunately, a lot of the perks of living in the 21st century actually disrupt the normal rhythms and functions of a healthy body. The food we eat, how we move our bodies, and the products we breathe in and coat our skin with all change the delicate communication patterns of our hormone-producing endocrine system.

The easiest and most influential way to support your hormones is through what you eat. There are seven specific hormones that communicate with your metabolic system, which is responsible, in large part, for regulating your weight.

A healthy metabolism can also protect you from a wide range of diseases that are thought to be weight and age-related, such as diabetes, heart disease, and cognitive decline, to name just a few.

You can reset a particular hormone in as little as 72 hours. Through a 21-day plan, you can target one hormone every three days to have your entire metabolic system running smoothly again.

Every three days, we'll help you understand specific hormones and how certain foods react with that hormone. By eliminating some foods and increasing your intake of others, you can help balance the production of that hormone in a "hormonal reset."

The hormones that are most commonly dysregulated in women, causing frustrating weight issues, include estrogen, insulin, leptin, thyroid hormone, growth hormone, and testosterone.

Over the next 21 days, you'll be able to stabilize each of these hormones without the use of drugs. By relying on delicious and nutritious foods to support your natural endocrine system function, your results will be fast and sustainable.

Unlike a crash diet, once your hormones are in balance again, simple life-long and enjoyable lifestyle changes can make the weight loss and other benefits permanent.

Resetting the Hormones in Your Life

If you're anything like many other women, you've tried everything else to lose weight. Calorie based diets don't work long-term. Spending hours in the gym is not only painful but unsafe and impractical.

The Hormone Reset Diet is only asking for a short, 21-day commitment to prove its long-term value to your life.

In three weeks, you can wake up feeling energetic, well-rested, and at the top of your game.

When you slip on your favorite jeans, you'll smile at how easy it is to do up the buttons. Your heart will fill with pride, and you'll hold your head higher as you strut down the street, knowing that you look healthier than you have in years.

When you get hungry, you'll reach for food that enhances your great mood, instead of comforting your depression. When a friend asks you to go out dancing or on a hike, you'll jump at the chance because, for the first time in forever, you have the energy, stamina, and desire to show the world what your body can accomplish.

Your boss will marvel at your productivity, and your significant other will tingle with anticipation as the sparks start to fly between you again.

Balancing your hormones won't only help you finally get rid of those infamous last seven pounds. It will help you get your life back.

During the 21-day reset, yes, some foods will be eliminated. But you'll discover that by looking for alternatives, you open up an entire world of new and exciting flavors. Boring and restrictive meals are a thing of the past. You're about to fall in love with food and your body.

You've spent too many weeks and years agonizing over your weight. Stop today. Start supporting your body's innate desire for balance, and you'll never want to return to your old habits again.

The Hormone Reset Diet is just the beginning. A healthy, happy, and long life is waiting for you, long after the 21 days are over.

Ready to get started?

Chapter 1:

What is the Hormone Reset Diet?

Understanding why this reset will work for you is an important part of the process to help you maintain your willpower and dedication throughout the next 21 days and beyond.

Hormones are responsible for much more than your teenager's mood swings and acne, or whether you'll be more likely to get pregnant in your 40s or start perimenopause.

We have over 50 different types of hormones that are responsible for regulating metabolism, sleep cycles, stress responses, growth rates of all kinds, and generally just keeping you alive by maintaining homeostasis in your body.

Your endocrine and nervous systems work together to send information throughout your body, triggered by both external factors, as well as need to keep the autonomic functions of your body operational at all times.

Your nervous system is lighting fast and transmits messages directly to cells for instant, short-lived responses. Your endocrine system, on the other hand, is more slow-moving, transmitting messages throughout your entire body using your blood.

Within your endocrine system, there is a collection of glands that make and secrete hormones. Some of these hormones do the work, and others delegate, simply acting as messengers telling another hormone what to do and when to do it.

Each hormone has a specific target cell type that it's able to communicate with through receptors on the cell. When a target cell is activated, the hormone either increases or decreases its function to keep your body homeostasis or balance.

If the receptors become damaged, the hormone can't effectively communicate with the cell, and processes inside of your body become confused and break down.

For women, there are seven hormones in particular that influence your metabolism and how your body decides to store or use energy. If these hormones fall out of balance, you'll be faced with weight gain and weight loss resistance, among many other frustrating and dangerous side-effects.

The 7 Hormones

If you can rebalance your hormones so that they're communicating with your cells and nervous system properly, your body will naturally regulate your weight. Humans are designed for efficiency, and holding on to unnecessary weight is anything but efficient.

The seven hormones we'll focus on throughout this 21-day reset are estrogen, insulin, leptin, cortisol, thyroid, growth, and testosterone.

Each hormone has its own chapter, which will explain in depth what proper function of the hormone should be like and how to get it back to normal. For now, let's take a quick look at the hormones you'll be working with.

Estrogen

Both men and women have estrogen, but it's particularly prevalent in women. It's responsible not only for a healthy reproductive system, but it also affects the heart and blood vessels, skin and hair production, and the health of your brain and bones.

Estrogen production is easily thrown out of order by our food and lifestyle choices, but high estrogen isn't the only problem. The key is to maintain a balance between estrogen and progesterone. As we age, our body naturally begins to produce less progesterone.

If estrogen levels are already high, the balance will just become more and more dysregulated over time.

An imbalance in your estrogen levels can not only lead to irregular menstrual cycles, but it is also closely linked to weight gain, particularly around the hips, thighs, and belly.

Insulin

Insulin is most well-known because of its role in diabetes. It's the hormone responsible for keeping blood glucose levels at a healthy balance, but, unfortunately, due to diet and lifestyle choices, insulin resistance or metabolic syndrome, has become one of the fastest-growing diseases on earth.

For many years, this condition was thought to be caused by obesity, but studies are starting to show that the reverse is actually true. Obesity is a symptom of insulin resistance. If you can rebalance your insulin levels by monitoring what you eat and when, you can stop your body from sending the signals to store more energy in fat, and start losing weight instead.

Leptin

Leptin is often called the hunger hormone because it's responsible for telling your brain when you have enough fat stored in your body to keep you safe and when you need to take in more energy.

If you have low body fat, your brain will throw out hunger signals to encourage you to find food. Unfortunately, if you have damaged leptin receptors, your brain will also continue to pump out hunger signals, whether you're actually in need of energy or not.

Hunger is very hard to ignore, and if your leptin levels are dysregulated, not only are you going to feel hungry constantly, but your body will also be actively trying to store any energy you consume as fat instead of using it immediately.

Cortisol

Cortisol is known as your stress hormone. When you've got too much on your plate and life is running you ragged, cortisol comes to the rescue...in a manner of speaking.

When your hormones are all well-balanced, and you're operating a relatively healthy body, cortisol helps to regulate your metabolism and immune response, among other important jobs.

When your stress response is triggered, cortisol is the hormone that shuts off operations of non-essential services. From your body's point of view, there's no point in worrying about digesting your food, keeping your ovaries healthy, or protecting your memory if your immediate survival is in jeopardy.

All your energy is diverted to systems that will keep you alive in the face of danger, such as your heart rate and getting enough blood and energy to your muscles.

This system is fantastic when you're actually in a life or death situation, but chronically elevated cortisol can lead to long-term digestive issues, immune disorders, mental health disorders, and much more.

Thyroid hormones

Thyroid hormones interact with a variety of other hormone pathways, and it's absolutely necessary to support a healthy metabolism. The thyroid hormone helps to regulate growth hormone, as well as your levels of progesterone, which all work together to regulate healthy body weight.

Genetic factors play a key role in thyroid hormone production; however, so does your gut health. Your thyroid is often targeted by autoimmune responses caused by what is commonly known as "leaky gut" syndrome.

When your immune system mistakes thyroid hormones for intruders, not only will inflammation and other immune responses start to create chronic damage in your body, but your thyroid hormones will also not be produced or received properly.

This can cause weight gain and retention, mood disorders, and a severe drop in energy levels, among other undesirable results.

Growth hormone

Growth hormone is responsible for stimulating the growth of nearly every tissue in your body, including your bones. With the right balance of this amazing hormone, you can actually grow your bones longer, instead of grinding them down over the years.

Of course, everything in this reset is focused on balance. While growth hormone is a good thing, too much of it can lead to fast growth and even enlarged extremities in extreme circumstances.

More common, especially in women, is the low production of growth hormone. In chronic conditions, this can lead to atrophied muscles and a decrease in bone density.

The growth hormone interacts with every other hormone your body produces. It helps to regulate the production of estrogen, insulin, and cortisol, and in turn, testosterone, leptin, and thyroid hormones keep growth hormone in check. Balance, on all accounts, is critical for overall healthy hormone function.

Similar to thyroid hormone, growth hormone is often mistaken for invasive proteins when your gut microbiome is in poor health. Autoimmune disorders caused by food sensitivities, particularly to dairy, in this case, can attack growth hormones, throwing your entire endocrine system out of sync.

Testosterone

Testosterone is a sex hormone that is found in higher concentrations in men but is still very important in women. Low levels have been linked to poor sex drive, but having too much can cause infertility.

It's not only concerned with your reproductive system, though. Testosterone helps to increase growth hormone and, together, they encourage lean muscle mass and fat burning. Without it, you can become resistant to weight loss, among other symptoms.

Men produce testosterone primarily in their testes, but women split the minute production between four different glands and tissues. This can be both good and bad. It helps to split the responsibility of maintaining the optimal balance between multiple players, but this can also cause a cascade of disruption between those same players.

As with all your hormones, balance is key.

A 21-day Hormonal Reset

Weight gain, fatigue, mood disorders, digestive struggles, and other uncomfortable *diseases* are your body's way of telling you something is wrong. It is not normal to feel unwell.

Many of these symptoms, especially for women, are signals that your endocrine system has a glitch. It isn't producing hormones effectively enough to manage your metabolism properly.

As we've already mentioned, the good news is that hormones are quick to reset themselves. Your body desperately wants to be in homeostasis, so if you can support its needs, it will gladly reset.

What a Reset Isn't

First and foremost, let's get clear on what a reset *isn't*.

A hormone reset isn't a cleanse. It's not a trendy detox or a quick fix.

It's not an easy button that will let you drop the last seven pounds so you can fit into your little black dress for one specific special occasion and then coast right back into your unhealthy habits.

A hormone reset isn't an overnight cure for metabolic diseases. For that matter, it isn't a *cure* for anything.

To be completely honest with you, this hormone reset isn't always going to be easy on you. You'll be asked to give up foods that you're chemically addicted to and some that you simply enjoy eating. You might experience symptoms of withdrawal, and some days you might feel worse before you start to feel better.

The next 21 days aren't all going to be pleasant. You'll be encouraged to support your dietary changes with lifestyle changes that might be out of your comfort zone right now.

But if you can commit to this hormone reset, and all its hard moments, by the end of it you will have naturally reset multiple systems in your body so that not only can you lose weight, but you'll also have more energy, better sleep, less stress and, overall, you'll get a lot more enjoyment out of the simple act of living each day.

What a Reset Is

It takes about 72 hours to clean your blood of excess hormones and bring it back into balance, so every three days of this reset, you'll be focused on a single hormone.

For the next three weeks, you'll systematically eliminate foods that are known to disrupt hormone production, and you'll add in foods that have been shown to help support your hormone production.

By resetting the hormones that are primarily responsible for your metabolism, you'll be able to finally coax your body into releasing any weight that is unnecessary—like those last seven pounds!

The best part of bringing your hormones back into balance is that when everything in your body is communicating clearly and all systems are operating well, you'll no longer be getting mixed signals from your body.

You'll get hungry when you need more energy, not when you're bored or emotional. You'll crave foods that make you feel alive, young, and energetic, and you'll have no trouble saying "no" to the heavy, bloating, guilt-inducing snacks of your past.

More Than Just a Diet

Studies have shown that weight loss, especially in women, is more effective when you control what you eat than when you focus on exercise. While there is some truth to the relationship between calories consumed and calories burned, contributing to weight gain, there is a lot more going on inside your body than simple mathematics. The quality of the calories you consume can be just as important as the quantity.

That's why this diet doesn't focus on numbers, but rather on the type of food you're eating, how you're eating it, and what your eating patterns are telling your body.

This type of diet can be supplemented by vitamins, but, more importantly, it can be supplemented by your mind and your movement.

Mindset

Editing your eating plan to become healthier and support balanced hormones isn't all about what you can't eat. It's just as much about what can eat and should be eating more of.

In cognitive-behavioral therapy, how a person *thinks* about a situation has a massive impact on how that person feels and reacts to that situation.

In other words, how you think about the food on your plate can have a greater effect on the way you enjoy it than the taste of the food itself. If you start this program focused on everything you have to give up, you'll make it impossible for yourself to appreciate all the incredible foods you're welcome to eat.

Instead, if you pay attention to the variety of flavors and beauty of the foods that you're encouraged to eat in abundance, you'll find yourself spoilt for choice throughout this program.

To help you keep a positive mindset throughout this process, and remind you why you've chosen to reset your hormones, you might find it useful to keep a journal.

You can use your journal to track your emotional ups and downs through the process, as well as your physical changes. Keeping track of your progress is a great way to stay motivated and determined to continue.

Make a note of how you feel before and after each hormonal reset, and any major changes you notice. While it may sound gross, you can even track your bathroom habits, making a note of how you digest different foods.

Throughout the next 21 days, you will be tempted to give up at some point. Having a really great reason to continue, and a few reminders of your progress might be the deciding factor in your desire to continue toward resetting your health.

You and your future health are worth it.

Physical Activity

As previously mentioned, your secret to losing weight is mainly dependent on the foods you're eating. But that doesn't mean exercise won't factor into the next 21 days at all.

Think of physical activity as a supporting role in your health. Without it, your results will be limited but, more importantly, if exercise isn't a part of your daily life, your long term health is guaranteed to suffer.

Luckily, the first few days of the reset will take exercise nice and easy, and the remainder of the program will be a slow yet steady intensity increase. The best news is that, if you follow the fitness tips recommended in <u>Chapter 11</u>, you won't be running for miles on end or spending hours upon hours in the gym. Instead, you'll be exercising more effectively to not only support weight loss but to make sure you keep the weight off long term and support healthy lean muscle and bone density for the rest of your life.

If you've taken the advice to start a hormone reset journal, you'll want to take a few key measurements before you get started so that in the end, you know exactly how far you've come.

Using a flexible measuring tape, jot down your measurements around your bust, waist, and at the fullest part of your hips and butt. If you tend to carry a lot of your weight in the lower half of your body, you can also measure each thigh. Similarly, if you're concerned about your arms, you can measure your biceps.

Of course, you'll also want to record your starting weight. It's a good idea to step on the scale first thing in the morning and just before bed the day before you start the reset.

By the end of the 21 days, your weight shouldn't fluctuate as drastically throughout the day, but before you begin, you could have a variance of five pounds or even more. It will be interesting to see how this fluctuation improves over time.

It's also a good idea to track physical symptoms like soreness, inflammation, headaches, etc. Ideally, over the next few weeks, you'll notice a steady improvement, but there may be times when the reset makes you feel worse before it makes you feel better. Making a note of any changes along the way can be motivating and enlightening.

The more you learn about your body now, the more power you'll have in the future to make tweaks to your lifestyle in the name of health.

Chapter 2:

21 Day Reset Preparation

The first and perhaps most important step in this process is to consult with your doctor or a nutritionist or dietician who is familiar with any current health concerns you may have. They will be able to provide more in-depth and personalized information, as well as answer any questions that might come up for you as you work your way through the reset.

If you don't have any preexisting conditions or a doctor that you see regularly, you may want to consider working with an integrative physician in your area. An integrative doctor is not only trained in conventional allopathic medicine but also understands and respects the body's natural ability to heal itself without prescription medications.

Working with a professional will help you fill in any micro-nutrient gaps you may have. Understand that it's very difficult to get 100% of the nutrition your body needs to truly thrive from food, both because of a lack of knowledge about what you need as well as a lack of availability.

You're probably incredibly effective at your trained profession, but if you're not an expert in hormone health, nutrition, physical fitness, *and* the intricate workings of the human body–that's okay!

Even if you knew everything about nutrition, there is to know, and you still might need to supplement it. Soil and produce quality are not what they used to be, not to mention location-based quality and availability.

With each hormone reset, you'll learn the most important vitamins and nutrients to support your hormone function, and if you feel the need to supplement, you'll have the option to do so.

From here on out, try not to obsess too much about every last detail. The more you focus on getting everything absolutely perfect, the more stressed you're going to get. As will become very apparent as you work your way through this book, stress is the enemy your hormones! Do what you can to the best of your ability, and let the rest take care of itself.

Nobody's perfect.

Adjust Your Eating Patterns

One of the reasons many women find following a strict diet helpful is because it tells you exactly what to eat, what not to eat, how much to eat, and sometimes even when to eat. Following orders for a short, set period of time leaves no room for mistakes.

But what happens when you go back to "real life?" Without the rigid structure of your diet, you fall right back into your old ways, and all the weight and disorders come right back.

With the 21 day reset, you'll have guidelines to help you understand what to eat and what to avoid, but it's not as restrictive as a standard caloric diet, and it naturally helps reset your eating patterns while it's working toward resetting your hormones.

By following this reset, you'll be establishing a new relationship with your meals. These new eating patterns will be easy to maintain long-term once you've developed a habit, helping to ensure your results are also long-term.

Respect Mealtime

While you do the reset, it's important that you practice structured mealtimes. Your hormones and nearly every other biological system in your body thrive off of routine.

By committing to three regular meals a day, eaten at relatively the same time each day, you'll be sending your body the message that it can expect to refuel at certain times, and there's no need to panic and start storing fat overnight.

On the other hand, if you train your body to expect food every two hours by constant grazing and snacking, it will want to be fed every two hours. Not only is this inconvenient, but it's also unsafe and dangerous to your health.

Digesting food is a lot of hard work, and your body needs time to get it done. Leaving 4 - 6 hours between meals and a minimum of 12 hours of overnight fasting will help your digestion keep up with its workload and run more smoothly.

You can also think about it this way: if you want your body to start burning fat, you have to give it the opportunity to do so. You need to stop eating all the time!

This is not just to reduce the availability of energy in the form of calories, but it's crucial to the regulation of hormones that tell your body when to store energy for times of need and when to *use* that stored energy.

Eat Real Food

One of the best things you can do for your overall health and certainly help rebalance your hormones is to move away from packages and toward whole foods, as close to their natural state as possible.

Throughout the 21 days reset, you'll focus on certain foods every three days, both to eliminate as well as to add. As a universal rule, you want to avoid processed, packaged, and pre-prepared foods as much as possible.

If you're budget and location allows, it's also important to choose organic foods to cook with. When it comes to meat, eggs, and dairy, choosing organic pasture-fed and finished, will make sure you're not ingesting a host of synthetic hormones that will mess up your progress.

Organic produce will protect you from hormone-disrupting toxins so, at the very least, have a look at the current "dirty dozen" and pick organic, local, and seasonal produce at every opportunity.

When you're grocery shopping, don't be fooled by marketing. Keep in mind that the food industry is a very lucrative business, but it is a business. Food producers want you to buy their food, and they'll say just about anything to trick you into eating more of what they have to offer. Just because something says, "natural" or "heart-healthy" doesn't mean it is.

When you cook from scratch, using whole food ingredients, you know exactly what you're eating, and you're eating in the way nature intended. Macronutrients, micronutrients, and fiber all work together in harmony when you eat whole foods rather than broken down, isolated pieces of food made in a laboratory somewhere.

Before you even get started, it's helpful to know and admit to your weaknesses. Create a chart for yourself that predicts which foods are going to call out to you when you're having a particularly rough day.

Create a "swap chart" for yourself. Identify foods that you constantly crave even though you know they aren't a part of a healthy diet. For example, your chart might have a column that lists ice cream, cookies, potato chips, fried chicken, and fast food.

Next to each of your weaknesses, write down a few options for swaps that you'll eat instead. Berries instead of cookies, popcorn instead of chips, and homemade, healthy freezer meals instead of fast food.

When you have an immediate and easily available alternative, you'll be much better prepared to avoid potential pitfalls.

Get in the Habit of Cooking

If you're buying real food for yourself and your family, you're going to have to get into the habit of cooking. A lot of people worry that cooking is too time-consuming, but with practice and strategy, home cooking can be faster and less expensive than eating out.

As with anything in life, the more you practice, the better you'll become.

Batch cooking and freezing food is one great strategy to implement. It's almost always more cost-effective to work in bulk, and cooking a larger batch of food doesn't often take much longer than cooking up a single serving.

You'll not only save time and money in the long run, but you'll be taking the guesswork and stress out of what to eat when time isn't on your side. Whenever you run up against a deadline, or feel under the weather or don't have time to cook for any other reason, instead of finding yourself tipping a delivery driver, all you'll have to do is take a look in your freezer.

Cooking itself can become a stress-relieving activity, bringing its own sense of joy an accomplishment to the table. Eating a delicious meal that you prepared is satisfying and something you can be proud of.

Spending more time hustling around your kitchen even adds up to more physical activity when compared to the alternative of sitting in your car as you go through a drive-thru. It may seem minor to you right now, but every minute you spend moving around instead of sitting has a dramatic impact on your hormonal health.

To help you flex your new cooking muscles, there is a collection of meal ideas at the back of the book to get you started. From breakfast, lunch, dinner, and even dessert, you'll have plenty of inspiration to get you through the next 21 days and well beyond.

Be prepared; these aren't recipes, but more like guides to helping you create your own unique recipes.

Get Back to Nature

Human bodies were not designed to spend 16 hours a day seated and another eight lying down.

They are pretty spectacular, though. As nature intended, our biological systems are self-healing, self-detoxifying, and designed to coordinate multiple systems in perfect harmony.

Unfortunately, because of our large and advanced capacity to think, human advancement has allowed us to deviate from nature in many ways.

We discovered how to modify and influence nearly every aspect of the human condition, from what we eat to how we sleep and move.

Just because we can process and modified foods to make them addictingly more palatable doesn't mean we should. Just because light bulbs and screens make it possible for us to lengthen our days and alter our sleeping patterns at will, doesn't make it healthy to do so. Finally, just because we don't have to chase our food down in a primeval hunt doesn't mean we don't need to find another way to move our bodies.

If you want to improve your health, one of the best things you can do is return to nature.

Circadian Rhythms

By definition, a circadian rhythm is "a natural, internal process that regulates the sleep-wake cycle and repeats roughly every 24 hours ("Circadian rhythm," n.d.)."

Following natural sleep patterns based on the rising and setting sun and regularized bedtimes allow you to spend more quality time in a deep sleep. Among other benefits, deep sleep increases the production of growth hormone, which, as you'll learn in <u>Chapter 8</u>, helps to regulate weight, particularly belly fat.

While you're on the Hormone Reset Diet, it's important to give your body as much opportunity to heal as possible. This means getting a minimum of eight hours of sleep every day and, if possible, up to 10 hours.

It can be very informative to keep your journal by your bed and make notes before you go to sleep, and when you wake up. Track the quality of your sleep, how well-rested you feel, how long it takes you to fall asleep, how tired you are at bedtime, stress levels, and general feelings at the end of the day and the beginning of a new day.

As you work your way through the 21 days, all of these metrics should start to improve.

The Great Outdoors

Unless you live in the middle of a highly polluted city, taking time each day to spend at least a half-hour outdoors every day can help reestablish the balance between serotonin and cortisol. Exposure to fresh air and sunshine gives you the opportunity to benefit from nature's ability to help you relax and get in a better mood.

Not all nutrients are taken in through food. Some are absorbed through your skin and from the air you breathe. Going for a walk in an area with plenty of trees improves the air quality and stimulates mental functions that can help protect your brain from cognitive decline.

When you get out into nature, use it as an excuse to unplug, leaving all your electronics at home. The physical movement, natural environment, and lack of immediate responsibilities will help you unwind. Focus on your breathing, find your own personal style of mediation, and simply appreciate the good things in life.

The boost of Vitamin D and oxygen helps to regulate your hormones and many other aspects of your overall health as well.

As little as 10 minutes can make a noticeable difference in your mood and energy levels, but dedicating 30 minutes a day to spend outdoors is ideal.

Manage Your Stress

Stress is getting blamed for just about every health disorder we can identify, and yet very little is being done actually to change or eliminate what causes us stress.

When it comes to stress and relaxation, sometimes the smallest things can make the biggest difference. You may not be able to quit your job, overcome your financial woes, or find yourself in the midst of the perfect family life, but you *can* work on your breath and meditation.

Both of these techniques are extremely powerful at reducing stress levels and, conveniently, they're both free, simple, can be done anywhere, at nearly any time, and only take a few minutes of your time.

There will be an entire chapter dedicated to cortisol, which is the hormone most closely related to stress. To help you prepare for this chapter, you should know upfront that you will be encouraged to eliminate caffeine from your diet during this reset completely. If you drink a lot of coffee, it is more than likely adding to your stress levels. It's a good idea to start reducing your consumption now, in preparation for Chapter 6, which begins on day 10 of your reset.

A good way to reduce reliance on caffeine progressively is to start cutting back and making strategic swaps at the same time. Depending on how many caffeinated beverages you drink daily now, try cutting that number in half, starting today.

Because sugar is just as addictive as caffeine, you'll also want to reduce the amount of sweetener you use in your coffee or tea. By the time you get to the cortisol reset, you will have already reduced or eliminated sugar, so removing caffeine should be much easier than you expect.

Every time you would normally reach for a cup of coffee or tea, replace it with decaf, green tea, or glass of water half the time. This will help you hydrate as well, which is a simple, non-hormonal way to keep your energy levels elevated.

On days three to five of the reset, try replacing all of your coffee with decaf and all your black tea with green tea or, even better, green tea.

For days six through eight, try to consume only green tea and non-caffeinated beverages. By day 10, you should be ready to wean yourself off of coffee completely.

Finally, exercise is a key component to relieving stress, though it isn't the main focus of this reset.

You should start incorporating movement into your days on a regular basis if you're not already. Chapter 11 covers recommended fitness efforts during the reset as well as after the reset and for the rest of your life. It might be helpful to read through that chapter before you start the program.

Breath Work

When you're in a state of stress, your body increases your heart rate, breathing rate, and blood pressure to give your muscles and brain the exact resources it needs to cleverly and speedily save your life.

The primary reason you breath is to absorb oxygen and remove carbon dioxide from your body. When you're stressed, you are more likely to take shallow breaths to get more oxygen into your body to aerobic power activity, like running for your life.

In nature's point of view, you cannot outrun a predator if you're taking deep, measured breaths. With that in mind, it should make sense that breathing deeply and calmly is a very effective "off" button for your stress response.

Breathing exercises help your parasympathetic system take over for your stressed sympathetic nervous system, reducing levels of cortisol in your blood, slowing your heart rate, and lowering your blood pressure, all thanks to a few deep, measured, and purposeful breaths.

Using breath work to reduce stress is that it only takes a few minutes, can be done anywhere by anyone, and it's completely free.

Meditation

Most people fall into one of two camps when it comes to meditation: you either love it or you hate it. Before you dismiss this section outright, try to understand the simplicity and the benefits of taking up this practice.

Meditation either uses negation or focus techniques.

The goal of negation is to clear your mind, leaving it blank. This allows you to release all of your cares and worries for at least a few minutes, giving you space to breathe easier and relax. When accomplished effectively, it can leave you in a state of semi-consciousness or even unconsciousness, similar to sleeping. If you can get to this point, you give your brain a chance to recover.

On the other side of the spectrum, focus

techniques encourage you to devote all of your attention to a single thought, feeling, or purpose. If you can master this technique, you will be better able to avoid distractions in all areas of your life.

Focus, for most people, is much easier to achieve than clearly your mind completely, and it can be used as a stepping stone for the more advanced negation practice.

If you have been finding that stress in your life is causing exhaustion during the day, when you need to be busy at work, which compounds your feeling of stress, a few minutes dedicated to focus will help you relax and pull your attention back to the task at hand. It stimulates wakefulness and can help you feel re-energized.

If stress is having a bigger effect on your sleeping patterns, a few minutes of guided meditations to help you clear your mind and leave the day behind you can help you get better sleep, improving your health in many ways.

Regardless of what kind of meditation you try, give yourself permission to be terrible at first. It's a skill that needs to be honed over time, but in just a few minutes a day, you should see noticeable improvements within a few weeks.

Chapter 3:

Estrogen

Estrogen is well-known as the hormone that gives a woman her feminine shape by filling out breasts and hips, but it triggers many other responses in the body as well.

We've talked about how important homeostasis is to health, and when it comes to estrogen, the ideal balance is found in a relationship with its hormonal partner, progesterone.

For instance, during a woman's menstrual cycle, estrogen is responsible for the growth of the uterine lining, whereas progesterone helps release it at the end of the cycle. They need to work together to ensure a complete, safe, and healthy cycle.

Cycles are a common theme in healthy biological systems. Along with balance, your hormones are very particular in the way they are used. For some processes occurring in your body, recycling is a great thing. Taking broken components of dead or damaged cells and turning them into healthy building blocks for new cells is what keeps your body youthful and in good working order.

Estrogen, however, is not meant to be recycled. Once it's produced, it's meant to be used as intended and then removed from your body.

Estrogen Dominance and Pollution

For most women, by the time you hit your 30s, your body starts to produce less progesterone, leading to estrogen dominance. To compound the problem, certain other hormones can upset the balance even further. Cortisol, for example, can block progesterone receptors, causing the ratio of estrogen to progesterone to lurch even further out of sync.

Not producing enough progesterone is only one-way balance is disrupted. A diet heavy in estrogen-laden foods, a stressful lifestyle, and a digestive system that doesn't effectively remove used up hormones and waste can also lead to disruptions.

Estrogen pollution is just what it sounds like—a build-up of estrogen that turns a healthy, essential hormone into a pollutant due to excess. Estrogen dominance and pollution is a long-term problem that doesn't happen overnight or because your balance is thrown off during one particularly stressful day.

When you've had too much estrogen coursing through your blood for too long, it can lead to weight gain, obesity, and cancer.

Doctors trained in the conventional medical system are taught to prescribe birth control medication to women under 50 who have any disorder that might be connected to an issue with estrogen. The added synthetic progesterone helps to balance out the estrogen.

After 50, women are assumed to be showing symptoms of menopause and will instead be prescribed hormone replacement therapy.

There may be a place and a time for prescription medications, but neither of these solutions actually *heal* your body, they simply mask your symptoms. A dietary reset can help balance your hormones naturally without a cascade of side effects.

Symptoms and Risks of Estrogen Dominance

If you've ever experienced breast tenderness or heavy, painful periods, your body has given you warning signs that your estrogen levels are getting too dominant.

47

PMS and mood issues are talked about as if they're a normal experience of being a woman, but, in reality, these are symptoms as well. Nothing about being in pain or discomfort should ever be considered *normal.*

If you'd like more scientific data about your own personal estrogen levels, getting regular PAP smears will help you, and your doctor notices any changes that happen over time.

Unfortunately, moodiness and sore breasts are minor symptoms of dysregulated hormones, but the development of cysts, resistance to weight loss, endometriosis, and even cancer are more severe and equally common symptoms.

Nobody likes to talk about breast cancer, but most women around the world live in fear of it. It's not a causeless fear, either. According to US statistics, one in eight American women will develop an invasive form of the disease at some point in her life (BreastCancer.org, 2019). If you balance your estrogen levels, you can play a part in decreasing that statistic by at least one woman.

Having too much estrogen floating around in your body is not a condition you want to take lightly. Thankfully, with a few tweaks to your diet and lifestyle, the power to reset your estrogen balance is in your hands.

Balance Estrogen Levels with Food

Before we start to rearrange the way you fuel your body, it's important to remember that the 21-Day Reset is just that, 21 days. You will not be forced to give up anything for the rest of your life, nor will you be forced to eat anything that you can't stand, making eating a miserable, joyless activity for the rest of your life.

When your hormones are in balance, the way your body reacts to food will change entirely. Estrogen is one of the first hormones we reset because it's very closely related to our relationship with food.

While most women don't think of being called "emotional" is a flattering compliment, it's also hard to argue the fact that women are more prone to what is called "emotional eating." That is, in large part, to estrogen. If we can balance this one hormone from the start of the program, our eating patterns will be much easier to manage throughout the rest of the program.

What to Eliminate and Avoid

The first two items you're going to eliminate from your diet for the next 21 days are probably going to be the most difficult and most beneficial: red meat and alcohol.

There are a lot of very popular diets and eating plans that support high meat consumption, and each of them has reasonable amounts of scientific data to back up their claims. Advising you to go meatless in the era of Keto, Paleo, and even Carnivore diets may surprise you, but please don't make any decisions until you've heard the reverse arguments first.

science

Meat eaters are simply more likely to have estrogen dominance, and that has been proven in multiple studies (Gottfried, n.d.).

Consuming animal protein also alters your microbiome and the varieties of bacteria that live in your gut. Having a healthy gut is a very popular trend right now, as it should be, and more evidence comes to light every day that shows a great deal of hormone regulation happens inside your digestive tract.

There is a subset of your microbiome, called the astrobleme, which directly affects your estrogen levels specifically.

Alcohol raises estrogen levels, and there's no good way to sugarcoat this fact. If you're struggling with your estrogen levels, alcohol will add to the problem.

It also slows down metabolism, further disrupts your astrobleme, raises cortisol levels, which, as we know, further disrupts your progesterone levels, and it challenges your sleep quality.

Your liver is a huge player when it comes to directing hormones through your bloodstream, and you probably won't be surprised to hear this, alcohol consumption wreaks havoc on your liver function.

Once your hormones are rebalanced, enjoying the occasional drink will not be overly detrimental to your health, but for the duration of this program, you'll want to avoid alcohol completely.

There is a very good chance that you'll feel and see a difference in your body within the first 72 hours of this plan, but it's crucial to keep the next 21 days free of all red meat and alcohol to really give your body a chance to recover. While estrogen might reset in three days, changing the flora in your gut takes longer but will be very beneficial to your overall success with this reset and your long-term health.

What to Enjoy More of

Since you won't be eating red meats like beef or pork, it's important to integrate alternative, clean proteins into your daily diet to keep your energy levels up. Some great sources of protein that will support healthy estrogen removal include:

- pastured poultry and eggs

- wild-caught, cold-water fish, especially salmon and sardines

- plant-based proteins such as quinoa, soy, buckwheat, legumes, nuts, seeds, especially chia & hemp seeds, and even algae like spirulina or chlorella

Finding the perfect balance of Omega 3 and Omega 6 fatty acids can help regulate your weight. A Standard American Diet (SAD) is disproportionately high in Omega 6s. By substituting processed food for salmon, sardines, and grass-fed butter, which are rich in Omega 3s, you'll be priming your body to burn fat instead of holding onto it.

Fiber is absolutely essential in helping your body remove waste. Studies have shown that 95% of Americans are deficient in this nutrient, which can lead to significant digestive issues, not to mention hormonal imbalances and a host of other chronic and life-threatening diseases (Quagliani & Felt-Gunderson, 2017).

Fiber-rich foods can help relieve symptoms of

bloating and constipation and get rid of excess estrogen in the process.

Too much fiber all at once can be hard on your system, though, so increase your consumption gradually, adding 5 g a day until you reach an average of 45 g per day.

It's surprisingly easy to increase fiber in your diet as it's present in all plant-based foods. Some of the highest quality sources include:

- chia, ground flaxseed, lentils, legumes, berries, and green veggies

All vegetables have fiber, but they're also incredibly nutrient-dense, providing your body with vitamins, minerals, and antioxidants it needs to stay healthy overall. For estrogen balance focus on getting great variety in the colors of your vegetables:

- leafy greens, broccoli, carrots, bell peppers, cauliflower, squash

There are those who very passionately argue against soy, citing studies that show how it is a major contributor to the increase in estrogen dominance related disorders and diseases.

And then there are others who reference studies done on Asian cultures, where soy-based products are consumed in high quantities even though estrogen-related disorders are extremely low.

For the purposes of this Hormone Reset Diet, soy can be consumed in moderate quantities, but the focus should always be on quality.

What some of the studies in the anti-soy groups fail to mention is that isolated soy compounds are heavily used in processed foods, such as protein powders, textured soy protein, and processed meat alternatives.

Another issue is that the vast majority of soy consumed is eaten by animals in conventional industrial farms. One of the reasons soy products are contributing to estrogen dominance is not because humans are eating too much soy, but because we're eating too much animal protein, which is consuming too much soy.

If you eliminate processed foods and conventionally raised meat from your eating plan, you'll not only significantly decrease the amount of soy you eat, but you'll also be automatically decreasing the amount of sugar, gluten, unhealthy fats, and synthetic hormones that you're consuming as well.

Finally, when you're eating foods in their whole form, as opposed to isolating specific compounds, you provide your body with more nutritional support to effectively digest and process the food.

If you choose to eat soy products, choose non-GMO organic options that go through as little processing as possible. Organic edamame, tofu, and tempeh are fantastic sources of clean, plant-based proteins, packed with vitamins and minerals that will help your endocrine system thrive.

.an, you'll not only significantly decrease the amount of soy you eat, but you'll also be automatically decreasing the amount of sugar, gluten, unhealthy fats, and synthetic hormones that you're consuming as well.

Finally, when you're eating foods in their whole form, as opposed to isolating specific compounds, you provide your body with more nutritional support to effectively digest and process the food.

If you choose to eat soy products, choose non-GMO organic options that go through as little processing as possible. Organic edamame, tofu, and tempeh are fantastic sources of clean, plant-based proteins, packed with vitamins and minerals that will help your endocrine system thrive.

Chapter 4:

Insulin

Your metabolic system relies almost exclusively on glucose to provide energy to all your major biological systems and organs. On the surface, this may sound like you have to provide your body with glucose in order to function continuously, but that is far from the whole truth.

In a healthy, perfectly balanced body, blood glucose levels hold steady at about 70 - 100 mg/dL. Carbohydrates are the easiest macronutrient for your body to break down into glucose. When you eat carbs, your metabolic system has easy access to glucose, which raises your blood sugar levels.

science

Understanding Insulin

When glucose in your blood increases, beta cells in your pancreas produce and release insulin. Insulin is the almighty hormone responsible for telling your body to move glucose out of your

science

bloodstream and into your adipose tissue for storage.

Before you start to blame every ounce of unwanted fat on insulin, it's important to recognize how important insulin is to your very survival. When blood sugar is chronically elevated, it can damage blood vessels, particularly those in your nervous system, heart, kidneys, eyes, and extremities, like your hands and feet.

Insulin is designed to protect against this kind of damage, while at the same time creating a backup plan for your future in case there comes a time when food is scarce.

Once enough, glucose has been moved out of your blood. Insulin production will shut down. If you don't reintroduce more food for an extended period of time, your blood sugar will continue to drop as your metabolic system continues to draw on that blood glucose for energy to maintain the normal operation.

If your blood sugar levels get too low, alpha cells in your pancreas trigger the production of glucagon, which tells your liver and adipose tissue to release the stored glucose back into your bloodstream.

If you continue to add new sources of glucose, however, your body will never need to tap into its stored energy and will instead continue to add to it with every new feeding.

Mediating Insulin Resistance

If your blood sugar levels are always high because you're constantly adding more glucose to your blood with constant snacking and grazing habits, your pancreas will be overworked, producing insulin to deal with the problem. At some point, there will simply be too much demand for insulin to keep up with, and your pancreas will start to fail.

Compounding this issue is the fact that if insulin is triggered too often, your body will stop responding to it properly. Sort of like the boy who called wolf, this is called insulin resistance, and if left unchecked can lead to Type 2 diabetes as well as a host of other health issues and consistent weight gain.

By regulating what you're eating and when, you can help support your body's normal insulin function, reestablishing the homeostatic relationship between insulin and glucagon.

Having too much insulin circulating in your bloodstream will also cause an increase in estrogen, which you learned about in the last chapter. This cascading effect can also lead to leptin resistance and a decrease in testosterone. Together, this combination of dysregulated hormones causes damage all over your body, steadily increases the amount of weight you gain, and is biologically incapable of losing.

Type 1 diabetes is not caused by diet or eating patterns, but rather it's a result of an underperforming pancreas. The pancreas simply does not produce enough insulin to regulate blood sugar properly and must be supplemented by externally administered insulin. Even with this in mind, choosing what and when you eat with care for your blood sugar levels can help regulate the disease more naturally though, to date, there is no cure for Type 1 diabetes, dietary or otherwise.

Balance Insulin Levels with Food

For many years, it was assumed that eating fat was the main reason for gaining fat. It's now understood that the problem is not with the fat you eat, but rather the sugar. When you're insulin resistant, your body stores glucose in fat cells, causing you to gain weight. To lose weight then, it makes sense that you'll want to eat less high-glucose foods.

Simple carbohydrates convert almost immediately to sugar in your bloodstream, and, of course, so does plain and simple sugar.

Your goal is to balance your eating plan and focus on dense nutrient options. If you severely restrict or eliminate all carbs from your diet, you can actually increase the production of reverse T3, which is the inactive form of thyroid hormone that blocks hormone receptors. You'll learn more about this in Chapter 8, but for now, suffice it to say some carbs are essential to your overall health.

At this stage in the reset, you want to pay attention to incorporating high-quality, healthy fats, clean proteins, and complex, slow metabolizing carbohydrates.

If you're planning on counting your carbs, keep in mind the fact that fiber, while considered a carbohydrate, actually passes through your digestive system without breaking down, so it isn't used as energy or raise blood glucose. When you look at the nutrition of a food item, net carbs are what will affect your blood sugar. To calculate net carbs, simply subtract the grams of fiber from the total carbohydrate count.

What to Eliminate and Avoid

Using the Glycemic Index (GI) to choose the food you eat is a useful way to understand how your food is going to affect your insulin levels.

High GI foods will convert to glucose more quickly, causing a corresponding spike in your insulin. Low GI foods take longer to break down and will have a more sustained effect on your insulin, without the undesirable spike and crash.

For the next three days, you're going to want to avoid foods that have a GI higher than 70. Some examples that are common in SAD include, but are not limited to:

- all added sugar and sweeteners, including white and cane sugar, honey, maple or corn syrup, and agave

- sugary drinks, including soda, energy drinks, sweet teas, and most fruit juices or punches

- Processed sweets like candy, cookies, chocolate bars, donuts, etc.

- white and whole wheat pieces of bread

- white rice, rice milk, and rice-based snacks like rice crackers

- sugared and processed breakfast cereals

- some fruits, particularly watermelon and very ripe bananas

- instant or boiled potatoes

Condiments and spreads like ketchup, bbq sauce, relish, and jam may show up as low or medium GI foods, but they are easy to eat in larger quantities than recommended, so be very conscious of your consumption of any pre-packaged sauces, dips, dressings or spreads.

When you're trying to decide what to swap your favorite soda or sweet treat for, don't assume you're making a healthy choice by opting for a sugar-free version. Artificial sweeteners can overstimulate your taste buds, making you even more attracted to sugary foods and causing you to find non-sweet foods distasteful. This is not natural and can lead to extremely disordered eating.

What to Enjoy More of

Slow releasing carbs are low on the glycemic index and generally come from whole food sources like plants that are also high in fiber. There are two types of fiber, and understanding the difference between soluble and insoluble fiber will take you one step closer to really understanding how your body processes the food you eat.

The soluble fiber, in its natural, unprocessed state, assists in the moderation of blood glucose levels. When it enters your digestive system and gets mixed with water, it thickens, becomes jelly-like, and sticks to the inside walls of your intestines.

The purpose of this is to slow your food down in the gastrointestinal tract, giving your digestive system more time to break it down into nutrients for use. This is why foods with high soluble fiber are lower on the GI because they take longer to convert to glucose.

Food choices that are high in soluble fiber and have low glycemic loads include:

- most fruits and vegetables, including avocados, pears, and stone fruits, Brussel sprouts, sweet potatoes, broccoli, and carrots

- legumes, such as black beans, kidney beans

- nuts and seeds, like flaxseeds, sunflower seeds, and hazelnuts

- some whole grains, particularly barley and oats

Insoluble fiber, on the other hand, doesn't slow food digestion. Instead, it adds bulk and weight to undigested waste, helping it move out of your intestines more efficiently, preventing constipation. It also helps to support the development of healthy bacteria in your gut microbiome, which has many benefits, both related and separate, to balanced hormones.

Insoluble fiber doesn't affect blood glucose levels, so even though it's great for digestion and health, it isn't as good of an indicator for food choices to regulate insulin specifically.

Additional Tips for Supporting Insulin

The more carbs you eat, and the more frequently throughout the day you eat them, regardless of quantity, the less likely your body will be to dip into its back up reserves. If weight loss is one of your goals, you want your body using the energy that is stored in your fat cells.

Some carbohydrates are necessary for health, but you're likely eating many more carbs than you realize at the expense of other important macronutrients like healthy fats and proteins. The most effective secret to reducing carbohydrates is to focus on eating whole foods and avoiding processed foods as much as possible, which is easier said than done, especially if you're dealing with a sugar addiction or are used to existing primarily off of premade foods.

Conquer Sugar Addiction

As with most addictions, a big part of overcoming your addiction is mindset and willpower. You must have a powerful reason for making a choice to "get sober" and stick to this commitment throughout all the withdrawal symptoms.

Sugar addiction is every bit as controlling as drug addiction. Sugar triggers a dopamine response, which is your body's natural way of providing you with a pleasant high for doing a good job at something. Unfortunately, the more sugar you eat, the more dysregulated your dopamine communication becomes, requiring a bigger "hit" to produce the same response.

Even if you don't consider yourself a sugar addict, if you've been eating a Standard American Diet for a significant amount of time, you're likely more dependent on your sugar high than you realize, thanks to the prevalence of simple carbs that convert quickly to glucose–like bread, pasta, and almost anything processed, sweet or not.

You'll need a strong mindset and a deep level of determination to kick this particular habit, but once you do, you will find that you feel great. You'll have more energy than you have in years, and you won't find yourself crashing nearly as often.

Get Comfortable in Your Kitchen

One of the best ways to clean up your carb intake is to start preparing your own meals from real, whole ingredients.

Almost everything that comes in a shelf-stable package has been tampered with in some way to make the food not only last longer but taste better. It's in the best interest of the food industry to get people addicted to eating. That's the best way to ensure they'll keep coming back for more, after all.

If you start cooking for yourself, you'll learn what foods are supposed to taste like, and your body will start processing them as nature intended.

Your taste buds play a significant role in your diet and your ability to maintain a healthy eating plan. It's normal to want to eat more food that tastes great and less food that you don't like.

What you might not realize, however, is that your taste buds could be lying to you.

A diet high in processed sugars, salts, and fats can damage your taste buds. They lose the ability to enjoy flavors that are healthy, getting confused by chemicals and additives.

Luckily, it doesn't take long to get your taste buds back to normal, and you can learn to like a wide variety of foods and flavors that you thought you would hate for life. To help this process along, you can try coaxing natural sugars out of vegetables by roasting them or adding healthy fats like olive oil or organic, pasture-fed butter.

By doing your own cooking, you'll develop a new relationship and respect for the food you eat, helping you adjust your mind as well as your hormones.

Chapter 5:

Leptin

Biologically speaking, the reason humans eat is to provide the body with the resources it requires to produce energy and keep all systems running efficiently. Under ideal circumstances, when you have enough power, you'll feel full. When you lack energy, your body will send out hunger signals to encourage you to eat again.

Unfortunately, for many different reasons, our bodies are rarely operating under ideal circumstances. For most of us, this means that we often feel hungry even when our bodies don't need more energy. If we eat anyways, we end up taking in more energy–or calories–than we need, so they get stored in our fat cells.

To a high degree, this frustrating cycle is caused by leptin or, more accurately, leptin dysregulation.

Leaning on Leptin

If you find yourself succumbing to hard-to-ignore cravings for food in the evening, even though you know you don't need any more energy, that is one very telling sign that you have an imbalance in your leptin levels.

One of the most interesting facts about this hormone is that it's released from fat cells, and therefore the amount of leptin produced by your body is directly related to the amount of body fat you have.

Leptin is your body's way of knowing how much body fat it has, which is an important biological safety net to keep you from starving during times of famine. When you have high leptin levels, your brain knows that you have adequate stores of body fat to keep you safe, theoretically setting systems in motion to allow you to eat less and burn more fat.

As your leptin levels decrease, your brain is signaled, and the systems reverse, causing you to eat more and burn less. Unfortunately, if the leptin receptors in your brain malfunction, your brain will continue to tell your body that it needs to consume and store more energy.

science

Leptin resistance is very similar to insulin resistance in that the more of this hormone that your body produces, the worse it's able to respond to it. The more energy you have stored in your fat cells, the more leptin is released, and the more resistant leptin receptors become.

Once again, we're faced with the reality that the problem is a hormonal imbalance that can't necessarily be addressed by the "eat less, exercise more" philosophy.

Consequences and Causes of Leptin Dysregulation

Anyone who has ever lost a considerable amount of weight because of a crash diet has probably also experienced the depressing effects of not only putting all the weight back on but actually even gaining more in the long-term.

You can thank leptin for this. When you lose a large amount of body fat in a short period of time, your leptin levels will drop dramatically, throwing your brain into a panic. The sudden lack of leptin signals danger and your brain will start screaming at you to eat more, and then it will take all the energy it can to refill the void in your fat cells.

Losing fat mass quickly on a calorically restrictive diet doesn't do anything to reverse leptin resistance, though, so even if you gain all the weight back, your hunger and storage signals won't turn off, causing you to pack on even more pounds.

If you lose weight by bringing your leptin hormones back into balance and healing leptin resistance, there won't be any reason for your brain to panic. Any weight loss will be gone for good, and as long as your leptin levels stay balanced, your weight will manage itself in the long-term.

The cause of leptin resistance is not 100% clear, but there are a few mechanisms that have been closely tied to the dysregulation of this particular hormone.

Chronically high leptin levels due to a high body fat index, as we've already discussed, is one clear culprit. Chronic inflammation also seems to be linked to the disorder, as well as having elevated levels of fatty acids in your bloodstream.

Balance Leptin Levels with Food

Everything about leptin acts as a one way street with two directions of traffic running through it.

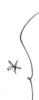

Triglycerides are the most common type of fat in your body. Any energy that you consume and don't immediately burn for fuel is converted to triglycerides for storage. High triglyceride levels interfere with leptin transportation to your brain, throwing your hunger signals out of a healthy range.

If you can avoid putting on fat, leptin will help you avoid putting on fat.

Inflammation is another system that both increases leptin resistance and is exacerbated by having too much leptin in our bloodstream. If you can't control your levels of inflammation, leptin will help you control your levels of inflammation.

The confusing feedback system of leptin only occurs when it becomes dysregulated. Properly balanced leptin is a key figure in maintaining homeostasis in your body.

What to Eliminate and Avoid

Foods that are highly glycemic and can lead to weight gain will disrupt normal leptin production, so balancing your insulin in the previous reset will help significantly, but you'll want to continue consuming mostly low GI foods throughout this reset as well.

Avoiding inflammatory foods is the main focus of the next three days.

Processed foods, plants in the nightshade family, and FODMAPS will all be removed from your diet for the rest of the program.

Ideally, you'll already have nearly eliminated all processed foods by now, but if you haven't yet, it's high time you say goodbye to anything fried and fast. Processed foods contribute to unhealthy gut bacteria, destroyed microbiome, autoimmune disorders, and inflammation.

Nightshades contain a chemical called solanine, which, in some people, interfere with enzymes in your muscles, causing pain and stiffness. They can also increase inflammatory response, irritating your gut and joints. Whether or not you know you have a sensitivity to these foods, it's a good idea to avoid eating them to give your body a few weeks rest. Foods in the nightshade family include:

- potatoes, tomatoes, aubergines, and peppers

FODMAPs are fermentable carbohydrates that don't digest well. These carbs don't get absorbed into your bloodstream, but instead, travel all the way to the end of your gut, where the majority of your bacteria live. Once they're here, the bacteria begin to eat them, which can be great for a healthy microbiome, but in a damaged gut, it can create gas, increased digestive issues, and lead to inflammation.

To reduce FODMAPs in your diet, avoid the following:

- Fructose, found in primarily in low GI fruits, especially canned fruits

- Lactose, a carbohydrate from dairy products

- Fructans, present mainly in wheat products but also in smaller quantities in onions, garlic, and bananas

- Galatians, found in legumes and pulses

Some vegetables are also FODMAPs, containing any one of the above compounds. High FODMAP vegetables to avoid over the next three days include:

- Asparagus, Brussels sprouts, cauliflower, artichokes, leeks, and mushrooms

What to Enjoy More of

Reducing carbs and FODMAP foods can put a dent in the types of foods you're used to reaching for, but it provides a great opportunity for you to get experimental with your food choices.

Throughout the next three days, you'll want to increase your intake of soluble fiber, which supports gut health and protects against obesity. Increasing sources of high-quality protein will promote weight loss and help bring your leptin levels back to their optimal functioning levels.

High fiber, low FODMAP choices include:

- leafy greens like kale, spinach, arugula, swiss chard, collard greens, and lettuce

- sprouts, carrots, zucchini, cucumber, kohlrabi, radishes, and squashes

If you eat fruit, look for wild or organic and/or stick to berries. Modern fruit is genetically engineered to have more fructose than nature intended, not only making it more addicting but also making it harder to digest.

High protein, low FODMAP choices include:

- organic tofu, tempeh, and edamame

- pasture-raised organic eggs

- nuts and seeds

Additional Tips for Supporting Leptin

One of the most effective ways you can reset your leptin is to burn more fat. Of course, that's easier said than done.

You've probably heard that muscle burns more energy than fat does, which is why those with leaner body mass indexes tend to have faster metabolisms. While you can't alter your current body composition instantly, you can alter what you're giving your body to break down.

High protein meals are harder to break down than carbohydrates, which puts your metabolism to work. After eating a high protein meal, your metabolism can increase by as much as 30% for as long as 12 hours (Wellness Resources, 2008).

By starting your day with a high protein meal, instead of a high carb meal, you're setting your metabolism on overdrive for the entire day. Because it takes longer to break down, you will also feel full for a longer period of time, making it easier to make it through the 5 - 6 hours before your next meal without falling victim to cravings.

Improve Your Sleep

Leptin follows a circadian rhythm, which means that levels are at their highest in the evening. The most effective time your body has to make repairs is at night while you're sleeping. By establishing a consistent bedtime for yourself, your hormones will be better adapted to increase at the appropriate time, rather than being confused by sporadic sleeping patterns.

Leptin helps your body burn fat for fuel instead of glucose, so anything you can do to help it work effectively will improve your chances of losing weight naturally. Getting a good eight hours of sleep every night, especially if you're trying to lose weight, is a great way to support leptin regulation.

To improve your sleep and help your body spend more time repairing when you aren't sleeping, don't eat after dinner. Ideally, you'll want at least a 12-hour fasting window between your last meal of the day and your first meal of the next day.

Digestion is a very complex process that requires a lot of work. While your body is working hard on digesting your food, it doesn't have the resources needed to perform other functions, like repairing the damage done throughout the day.

If you eat your last meal 3 - 4 hours before you go to sleep, the vast majority of your digestive process will be complete, giving your body a full eight hours to do as much repair work as possible while you sleep.

Adapt to Intermittent Fasting

Giving your body a 12-hour window of fasting overnight is considered a low-intensity form of Intermittent Fasting (IF).

The longer you give your body to digest your food before giving it more work to do, the better your metabolic system is able to manage triglyceride levels better. Remember, a buildup of triglycerides can lead to leptin resistance.

Allowing enough time to fully digest your food before you eat again forces your body to start finding energy that is roaming through your bloodstream, not only preventing the excess energy from collecting in your fat cells but also helping your body more efficiently burn through excess fat that has already been stored. All in all, good digestion and fewer feedings per day helps you lose weight.

Constant grazing and snacking throughout the day can also affect insulin sensitivity, not only dysregulating multiple hormones but also causing you to eat more than you need to.

Instead of stressing yourself by counting every calorie you consume, simply try to avoid large meals and stop eating when you're not quite full.

We've talked about hormone cascades and how they take time to work through your bloodstream. For this reason, it can take 10 - 20 minutes for your hunger hormone, leptin, to completely turn off once you've ingested enough energy. If you eat until your 80 - 90% full, you'll more than likely find that after a short rest, you feel completely satiated. By eating your meal slowly, savoring each bite, you'll not only help your digestive system better process your food, but you'll also give your hormones more time to adjust your hunger signals properly.

Chapter 6:

Cortisol

Cortisol has a rather infamous reputation as the stress hormone. It's one of the hormones produced by your adrenal glands, and when it's running rampant through your bloodstream, this hormone can be the cause of significant damage.

But it's not just a villain.

Cortisol plays an important part in your overall health and safety as well, if it's properly balanced. We all need this hormone to help us cope in crisis situations, but it's important that we're able to effectively manage the hormone so that our body has time to relax and isn't always trying to put out fires.

The Good Side of Cortisol

There are four layers to your adrenal glands, each one producing a different hormone.

Epinephrine and norepinephrine, also known as

adrenaline and noradrenaline, is responsible for the fight or flight response. It's controlled by your sympathetic nervous system (SNS) in a closely coordinated relationship with what is called the Hypothalamic-Pituitary-Adrenal Axis (HPA Axis).

The rest of the hormones produced by your adrenal glands are triggered through a hormone cascade that begins in the HPA Axis.

When you experience stress, your SNS activates adrenaline, which, in turn, speeds up your heart rate and begins to direct blood away from your digestive system and toward your muscles.

At the same time, a cascade of hormones trickle down from your hypothalamus to your pituitary gland, and finally to the adrenal cortices on top of your kidneys, triggering the release of cortisol.

Day to day, these hormones balance our blood sugar and blood pressure, but during a stress response, cortisol increases blood pressure, pumps glucose into your bloodstream, and shuts down non-emergency systems like digestion, immune response and reproductive development.

Once these stress hormones saturate your blood, eventually, your hypothalamus will get the message and want to reestablish homeostasis in your blood. It will stop producing the hormone that started the entire cascade, slowly but surely shutting down the stress response.

The Dangers of Excessive Cortisol

You've no doubt heard of the fight or flight response and how early humans needed this to survive from attacks of saber tooth tigers. As true as that may be, there aren't too many tiger related high-speed chases in the world today, but in 2006, a Canadian woman did wrestle a polar bear that was advancing on her son and his friend. She won that fight, thanks to a little help from the hormone partnership between adrenaline and cortisol (Waldie, 2018).

Unfortunately, if these super-human hormones stay elevated all day, every day, it can cause a number of problems.

The really tricky issue with cortisol is that it lingers in your blood until the hormones are broken down by enzymes, which can take some time. The longer cortisol stays in your bloodstream, the longer your digestive system, reproductive system, and immune response are turned off.

Because it dysregulates your digestive system, it can wreak havoc on your gut health and microbiome. Chronic high cortisol levels contribute to weight gain, specifically around your belly, where there is four times the number of cortisol receptors.

It should help you feel more alert to your immediate surroundings, but it shuts off brain function related to memory and has been linked to Alzheimer's disease and other permanent cognitive issues. It's been known to accelerate the aging process in other ways as well, contributing to muscle loss, a decrease in collagen, and even osteoporosis.

Another hormone that we're going to look at more closely in a few chapters is the growth hormone. The growth hormone helps to balance cortisol. The more growth hormone, the less cortisol, and vice versa. Unfortunately, as we age, we start to produce less growth hormone, and cortisol levels are thrown even further out of balance.

Balance Cortisol Levels with Food

Since a huge majority of people are suffering from an extreme excess of this particular hormone, for the rest of this reset, your goal is to reduce cortisol as much as humanly possible.

There are many lifestyle factors that relate to cortisol production, but taking stimulants to help you keep up with the stress of daily life can actually compound the damage stress itself does to your body.

What to Eliminate and Avoid

The two most common stimulants used in the 21st century are caffeine and sugar. Since we've already addressed sugar in resetting your insulin, it's time to talk about coffee.

Caffeine, which actually includes teas, energy drinks, soda, and even chocolate, can be a really effective stimulant when used in moderation. If over-consumed, it can overstimulate your nervous system, leading to exhaustion. This can result in anxiety, heart palpitations, and disrupted sleep.

Two factors that you'll see recurring often in

relation to your overall health is stress reduction and high-quality sleep. Caffeine sabotages both of them.

The health effects of coffee have been debated for generations, with no clear winning side. Some experts tell you to drink as much as possible because it's the largest source of antioxidants for most Americans.

Others will tell you that it can lead to cancer.

If you're following the recommendations of this reset, you'll be eating plenty of richly colored vegetables, so you shouldn't need coffee to serve as your antioxidant solution. And if you can get your hormones under control again, you should have to be concerned about coffee giving you cancer either.

But for at least the next three days, and preferably until the end of this reset, you will learn how to survive without artificial stimulation. The truth is, you shouldn't need stimulation to stay energized throughout the day, that is what calories, combined with quality sleep, are for.

Artificial stimulation of your hormones confuses the normal process of communication within your body, and our goal throughout this program

Chapter 8:

Growth Hormone

The growth hormone is linked very closely to the aging process. Starting in your 30s, your body starts to produce less growth hormone naturally.

Among other responsibilities, growth hormone helps to balance cortisol. The more growth hormone your body produces, the lower your cortisol levels will be. As you produce less growth hormone, you not only have to deal with the immediate results of this deficiency, but you also have to cope with even more dysregulated cortisol.

How Growth Hormone Works

The growth hormone is produced directly in your pituitary gland, triggered by stimulating hormones produced by your hypothalamus.

There are five main factors that stimulate the production of GH:

1. high amino acid levels in the blood
2. low blood glucose/hypoglycemia
3. low fatty acids in the blood
4. healthy stressors
5. exercise

Once stimulated, the growth hormone goes to work, trying to balance out the first three stimulating factors with a goal of lowering amino acid levels in your blood and increasing blood glucose and fatty acid levels.

Some of the hormones will bind with target receptors on your liver and eventually gets converted to Insulin-like Growth Factor 1 (IGF-1).

IGF-1 promotes protein synthesis by binding with receptors on your skeletal muscle cells, encouraging the absorption of amino acids, balancing out the first stimulating factor.

When amino acids link together, they create proteins. Since this is specifically happening inside your muscle cells, the new amino acid chains increase the size of the muscle and improve function.

When the growth hormone interacts with your liver, it stimulates the process of

Additional Tips for Lowering Cortisol Levels

Of course, when it comes to non-edible factors, it's important to stress once again just how big of factor *stress* plays in a healthy balance of cortisol production. Taking away caffeine can be a significant stressor for many people, so you'll need to find ways to compensate.

Supplementation of key nutrients and minerals can be a big help, but so can further stress reduction techniques.

Supplements

Your goal should be to stimulate your metabolism, giving you the energy you need without stimulating your nervous system, making you jittery, and increasing your stress response.

Several studies suggest that B-vitamins can help inhibit cortisol and reduce symptoms of stress, particularly in women (Stachowitz & Lebiedzinska, 2016).

A high-quality B-complex supplement will give you a specially formulated combination of the potent vitamins, but you can also incorporate it naturally into your diet by using nutritional yeast.

Nutritional yeast has been used as a nutrient-dense flavoring agent for potentially thousands of years, but as a vegan diet has continued to rise in popularity, so has this unique fungus.

A single serving of nutritional yeast can provide up to 9g of protein as well as a significant portion of your recommended daily intake of Vitamins B-1, B-2, B-6, and B-12.

It has a somewhat nutty or cheesy flavor and is commonly used in dairy-free cheese alternatives.

Approximately 50% of Americans are deficient in magnesium, which happens to be a mineral that is involved in a cyclical relationship with cortisol (American Osteopathic Association, 2018).

Your body needs magnesium to respond to stress effectively, but cortisol depletes magnesium. To add to the problem, you need magnesium to absorb Vitamin D properly, which is another vitamin that has been shown to have positive effects on regulating cortisol.

Supplementing with magnesium, or at least eating plenty of magnesium-rich foods, is a great way to help balance cortisol. Green leafy vegetables, nuts, seeds, legumes, and cold water fish are good food sources.

Vitamin D is available in the supplement form as well, but it can also be soaked in through your skin with 15 -20 minutes of careful sun exposure each day.

Finally, a family of non-toxic plants called adaptogens can come to your rescue. These herbs have been used for centuries in ancient holistic healing techniques like Ayurveda and Chinese medicine, but they are resurging in popularity in popular culture. Though trendy does not always correspond to effective, in this case, it makes a very healthy selection of herbs more accessible to the public.

Adaptogens help your body adapt and deal with all varieties of stress.

Your body is designed to respond to muscle damage by making your muscles stronger. There is a growing body of evidence that suggests adaptogenic herbs can do the same thing, but for your adrenal glands. Instead of stress making you weaker and more vulnerable, your body will learn to respond more quickly and effectively with unavoidable exposure to stress.

Some supplements to look for include:

- ashwagandha, Holy Basil, licorice root, robiola, ginseng, and decaffeinated matcha

Stress Reduction Techniques

Oxytocin is sometimes called the "love hormone" because it's released when you're involved with social bonding. Hugging, laughter, and even cuddling your dog can release this hormone, which reduces the effect of stress.

Part of your challenge over the next three days, and hopefully for the rest of your life, is to schedule more time for social fun and enjoyment.

Getting your body moving is another great way to reduce cortisol levels, but you need to focus on calming, relaxing activities. Extreme exercise is actually going to increase cortisol further, whereas a leisurely walk out in nature for 20 - 30 minutes a day will do a lot more for your stress levels.

You might also want to try barre classes, Pilates, yoga, or an easy jog. The key is to find an activity that you enjoy doing that will help you relax. Encouraging friends to join you will maximize your stress reduction.

We talked about meditation and breathing techniques in Chapter 2, and if you haven't started practicing these yet, now is the time. Breathing exercises and meditation can help drastically reduce stress, lowering your cortisol levels significantly.

Some research has even shown that shallow breathing through your mouth while you can increase cortisol, so taking some time before bed to simply take in deep breaths through your nose can improve sleep quality and reduce stress.

Leptin and growth hormone regulation also require high-quality sleep, so relaxing before sleep helps on multiple levels.

Insulin-like growth factor (IGF-1) is very similar to growth hormone, but it's produced by your liver. It regulates fat burning and blood sugar levels when you're not eating–such as when you're sleeping.

Controlling your thoughts to avoid increasing stress before you fall asleep can be hard to do, as it's often a time when we start to reflect on the day we just finished and the one that is on its way. Practicing meditation can help stimulate a relaxed, peaceful, and healing mind to help you fall into a deep, restorative sleep.

Chapter 7:

Thyroid Hormones

Your thyroid is located in front of your trachea in your neck, and it's responsible for producing three key hormones: triiodothyronine (T3), thyroxine (T4), and calcitonin.

When we refer to thyroid hormones in the future, we're talking specifically about T3 and T4. Thyroxine, T4, is more prevalent in a hormone, but it's also weaker. T3 is about four times more potent, but a healthy, well-functioning endocrine system has the ability to convert T4 to T3, increasing effectiveness overall.

These hormones help regulate homeostasis in your body that, by now, you should understand your body's preferred condition. Maintaining optimal body temperature, skin moisture, blood pressure, digestive juices, and level of oxygen, calcium, and cholesterol in your blood are just a few of the tasks on your thyroid's to-do list.

We talked about the HPA Axis in relation to the

production of cortisol, and a very similar system is responsible for the production of thyroid hormones, only now we're dealing with the Hypothalamic-Pituitary-Thyroid Axis (HPT Axis).

The cascade of hormones begins when homeostasis is thrown out of whack for one reason or another, and turn off again with negative feedback. Once there's too much thyroid hormone running through your blood–not being used–your hypothalamus and pituitary gland will sense it and stop stimulating the thyroid.

When you have a hormonal imbalance, your thyroid might not turn on and off appropriately.

Symptoms of Thyroid Dysfunction

Thyroid hormones that are doing their job properly will stimulate your appetite and digestion, enabling the breakdown of nutrients so they can be absorbed and put to work. Almost every cell in your body has receptors for thyroid hormones, so you can just imagine how vital these particular hormones are to your overall health.

There are two main types of thyroid conditions: hyperthyroidism, which occurs when your thyroid produces too many hormones and hypothyroidism, which happens when it's not producing enough hormones.

Hypothyroidism typically causes slow metabolism, respiratory, and cardiovascular activity. This can translate to symptoms of fatigue, weight gain, hair loss, heavy menstrual cycles, constipation, and possibly feeling cold all the time.

A low functioning thyroid is thought to be caused primarily by either iodine deficiency or an autoimmune disorder called Hashimoto's thyroiditis.

Your thyroid cannot produce hormones without iodine. In fact, thyroid function is the only known use for iodine, but it's an important one.

A deficiency of this mineral will cause your thyroid to swell as your HPT Axis continues to direct trigger hormones to your thyroid, even though it can't keep up with the demand. The hormone cascade effective gets stalled, pooling excess trigger hormones into your thyroid, where they collect with nowhere to go. This can cause what is known as goiter and results in a sensitive, swollen lump in your neck.

On the opposite end of the spectrum, we find Hyperthyroidism or an overactive thyroid that produces too much thyroid hormones. This increases metabolism as well as respiratory and heart rates beyond safe levels. Unstable weight loss, insomnia, irritability, diarrhea, and heat intolerance are symptoms of an overactive thyroid.

Another autoimmune disorder, Graves' disease, is the most common cause of hyperthyroidism.

Autoimmune Disorders and Thyroid Hormones

Autoimmune diseases occur when the immune system starts to attack itself. When it's thyroid dysfunction in question, the body specifically destroys your thyroid, making it unable to respond to the need for thyroid hormones effectively.

In the case of hyperthyroidism, your immune system produces an antibody called thyroid-stimulating immunoglobulin (TSI), which mimics the trigger hormone produced by your pituitary gland in the HPT Axis cascade. Unfortunately, TSI does not turn off when there is enough thyroid hormone in your bloodstream, but it continues to trick your thyroid into thinking it needs to produce more hormones to maintain homeostasis.

There are prescriptions and surgeries that can help manage symptoms of autoimmune disorders and the resulting thyroid dysfunction, but these solutions won't heal your body. By addressing the root cause of the disorder, you can reset your thyroid hormones to function properly.

Before we move on, it's important that you understand that there's a difference between rebalancing your hormone levels in 72 hours and curing an autoimmune disorder. The foods you do or do not eat can certainly help start the process of healing your gut, but that kind of damage takes time to repair. This reset does **not** claim to heal or cure any diseases that you may be suffering from.

One of the areas that your thyroid hormone is very active is in your gastrointestinal (GI) tract. Thyroid hormone controls glandular secretions, specifically alkaline and intestinal fluid, that help the smooth muscle surrounding your GI tract move waste out of your body.

If you have too much T3 circulating, it can result in diarrhea. Too little, and you'll be constipated. Both of these conditions can affect the bacteria that live in your gut.

When food doesn't break down and move out

properly, it can create micro holes in your intestinal tract. Undigested food particles and proteins can sneak through these tears into your bloodstream, causing an autoimmune response. This is commonly known as "leaky gut syndrome."

In yet another disturbing cycle, dysregulated production of thyroid hormone can increase your chances of developing an autoimmune disorder, and autoimmune disorders are one of the primary culprits for dysregulating thyroid hormone.

Balance Thyroid Hormone with Food

In the US, hypothyroidism is more common than hyperthyroidism, which means that the balance is more commonly due to a lack of thyroid hormones. That being said, it's not uncommon to vacillate between the two conditions, similar to the highs and lows of blood glucose levels.

To help your body naturally reset to the appropriate balance of thyroid hormones, the thyroid itself needs to be supported. In other words, instead of trying to influence how much hormone is being produced, we want to support the gland itself so that it can better regulate its own production in the long term.

What to Eliminate and Avoid

You may have focused in on the need for iodine in thyroid function. Worldwide, iodine deficiency is the leading cause of hypothyroidism, but it's extremely rare in the US, so using your thyroid as an excuse to eat more salty snacks is not going to solve any problems. Paying attention to how much iodine you're ingesting is a good idea, though, because you don't want to confuse your thyroid by having too much.

Goitrogens are foods that block iodine absorption. Raw cruciferous vegetables and soy are the most common culprits. These vegetables can still be amazingly powerful for your overall health, and even balancing multiple hormones, but you'll want to steam them during the reset.

Beyond iodine regulation, there are certain food items that are known to be thyroid disruptors. In other words, they suppress thyroid function.

The first food item you're going to want to completely remove from your diet for the remainder of this reset is gluten. You may or may not have a sensitivity to gluten, but that isn't actually what is causing the problem in this case.

The proteins in gluten mimic the proteins that are in your thyroid. If you happen to have an autoimmune disease, which often remains undiagnosed, your immune response is going to be triggered every time you consume gluten.

Not only is this going to continue to damage your thyroid, but it will also trigger an immune reaction throughout your body, worsening symptoms of inflammation, fatigue, and more.

Refined and processed grains, even those that are gluten-free, can cause similar immune responses due to similar proteins.

For best results, you want to stay far away from all of the following:

- bread, breakfast cereals, wheat, rye, barley, oats, millet, rice, spelled, etc.

Remember, you don't have to be gluten-free for the rest of your life, just long enough to reset your hormones and, if necessary, heal your gut.

Peanuts can also negatively disrupt your thyroid. They're not only goitrogens but also extremely acidic and inflammatory, and have been known to kill the good bacteria living in your gut. Your microbiome is crucial to a healthy immune response, so it's time to eliminate peanuts from your diet.

What to Enjoy More of

Eliminating gluten products from your diet can be a very difficult adjustment for most people who are used to the Standard American Diet (SAD). Before you go out in search of highly process gluten-free alternatives that are just going to add a lot of chemicals and toxins to your diet, consider sprouted grains and coconut flour products as a healthier alternative.

When grains are sprouted, their protein structure changes enough that your immune system shouldn't confuse them for thyroid hormones. The process of sprouting also kills off phytic acid, which allows your body to better absorb the nutrients from the grain, instead of storing them as fat (DoctorOz, 2014).

Next, if you're concerned that you can't even trade your favorite lunchtime sandwich in for peanut butter on celery, don't panic. You can still eat just about any other nut butter of your choice, but almond butter will have the most benefits. Almonds have a good supply of the amino acid L-arginine, which increases growth hormone, which we'll talk more about in the next chapter.

To support healthy gut bacteria, you'll want to get a good variety of fruits and vegetables that are high in fiber, which provide plenty of fuel for the good bugs in your stomach. Eating plenty of raw vegetables is great, but be sure to cook any cruciferous vegetables like broccoli and cauliflower.

For proteins, pasture-raised organic poultry and eggs are great for thyroid support, as is seafood. In fact, all high quality, organic pasture-fed meat can be healthy for those suffering from hypothyroid and gut health but wait until the end of the reset to add red meat back to your diet.

Probiotic foods are also incredible for your gut health. Some great choices can be:

- Fermented foods like kimchi, sauerkraut, pickled vegetables, tempeh, and miso

- Fermented beverages like kombucha, water, or coconut kefir

Once the 21-day reset is complete, you can also try adding in cultured dairy products like yogurt, buttermilk, and milk kefir. Some types of cheese are also probiotic, but look for labels that say "live" or "active cultures."

Raw nuts are also great for gut health, especially Brazil nuts. They're high in selenium, which is known to support your T3 and T4 production in your thyroid.

Additional Tips for Healthy Thyroid Function

Women are highly over-represented in statistics of thyroid dysfunction, being ten times more likely than men to develop hypothyroidism (Vanverpump, 2011).

Diet can have a major impact on your thyroid hormone production, but when you take into consideration what a close relationship it has with growth hormone and your sex hormones—estrogen, progesterone, and testosterone—it's a great idea to support this hormone in many ways as possible.

Understanding how your genetics factor into your thyroid health, as well as how you can influence those genetics in your favor, is important, as is avoiding as many environmental toxins and stressors that might have a negative impact on your genetics is also an effective way to be proactive about your future health.

Genetics and Epigenetics

Many health disorders seem to run in the family, and that's often because of our genetics. Thyroid disorders are one of these potentially hereditary health disorders. But blaming unbalanced thyroid hormones entirely on your genetics is not only an incomplete truth, but it's also defeatist and unhelpful.

While you may have a genetic predisposition to poor thyroid health, your DNA doesn't have to have the final say.

Epigenetics can also help you determine and self-regulate your own fate.

Your genes can exist in your body in either an activated state or a deactivated state. If a gene is deactivated, it won't cause the disruption that it's potentially capable of.

Factors outside your genetics influence whether or not your genes get turned on. Even if every woman in your family has been diagnosed with thyroid disorders, there is still hope that your own personal disorderly genes will never get turned on.

What kind of factors influences your epigenetics? Diet, exposure to chemicals and environmental toxins and stressors, physical fitness, social experiences, trauma, and some medications.

If you find this hard to believe or accept, think about identical twins. They have the exact same DNA and genetics, but over time, they become more and more individualized as they each interact differently with their environment, activating or deactivating certain genes in different ways.

A positive note in relation to epigenetics is that once a gene is turned on—or off for that matter—it doesn't necessarily have to stay that way.

A healthy diet, regular physical activity, and low exposure to contaminants can help your epigenetics return to their optimal health-inducing state.

Environmental Toxins and Stressors

With your genetics in mind, there are a few specific environmental toxins and stressors that have been known to influence how your thyroid hormones get expressed.

First of all, severe carb restriction can increase reverse T3 production, which blocks thyroid receptors.

T3 is the active form of thyroid hormone that boosts your metabolism and stimulates the use of fat in your cells for energy. Reverse T3 is the inactive form, which doesn't just mean that it's "off," it also works against your metabolism, stopping your fat-burning potential.

Because your thyroid requires iodine, which is a halogen, as well as selenium, which is a metalloid, to function properly, it is particularly susceptible to damage from similar, yet harmful, halogens and heavy metals. Industrial chemicals, herbicides and pesticides, toxins in beauty products and other household commodities, and heavy metals can severely damage your thyroid.

We'll talk more about how to mitigate the effects of environmental toxins in Chapter 9.

Finally, your thyroid is also sensitive to disruptions in your other hormones, such as estrogen and testosterone, leptin, growth hormone, and cortisol. If you're one of the many women suffering from a thyroid disorder, committing to this reset will help from multiple angles.

Chapter 8:

Growth Hormone

The growth hormone is linked very closely to the aging process. Starting in your 30s, your body starts to produce less growth hormone naturally.

Among other responsibilities, growth hormone helps to balance cortisol. The more growth hormone your body produces, the lower your cortisol levels will be. As you produce less growth hormone, you not only have to deal with the immediate results of this deficiency, but you also have to cope with even more dysregulated cortisol.

How Growth Hormone Works

The growth hormone is produced directly in your pituitary gland, triggered by stimulating hormones produced by your hypothalamus.

There are five main factors that stimulate the production of GH:

1. high amino acid levels in the blood
2. low blood glucose/hypoglycemia
3. low fatty acids in the blood
4. healthy stressors
5. exercise

Once stimulated, the growth hormone goes to work, trying to balance out the first three stimulating factors with a goal of lowering amino acid levels in your blood and increasing blood glucose and fatty acid levels.

Some of the hormones will bind with target receptors on your liver and eventually gets converted to Insulin-like Growth Factor 1 (IGF-1).

IGF-1 promotes protein synthesis by binding with receptors on your skeletal muscle cells, encouraging the absorption of amino acids, balancing out the first stimulating factor.

When amino acids link together, they create proteins. Since this is specifically happening inside your muscle cells, the new amino acid chains increase the size of the muscle and improve function.

When the growth hormone interacts with your liver, it stimulates the process of gluconeogenesis. Remember, it was called as a response to low blood glucose levels, so now it wants to rebalance them. The hormone binds to receptors on adipose tissue, activating an enzyme called hormone-sensitive lipase. This starts to break down triglycerides that are stored in your fat cells into glycerol and fatty acids.

This process effectively raises blood glucose and fatty acid levels while it burns fat. Adequate levels of growth hormone can really come to your aid when you're trying to lose weight.

When IGF-1 interacts with your bones, it increases bone deposition and resorption, helping your bones grow thicker and stronger. It also works inside your cartilage, encouraging interstitial growth, or lengthening.

As you age and produce less growth hormone, your bones can become more brittle, and your cartilage depletes, reducing mobility and stability of your bones.

Signs and Causes of Growth Hormone Imbalance

The Hormone Reset Diet is primarily concerned with balance. You don't want too much or too little of any hormone, and you want your body's natural functioning to be able to discern and produce exactly the right amount when, and only when it's needed.

Low growth hormone production can lead to mood changes like anxiety, minor depression, and general feelings of unease. If you're not producing enough growth hormone, you'll likely feel fatigued and probably have issues with weight gain.

Many of the so-called "normal" signs of aging are also symptoms of low growth hormone.

Growth hormone deficiency is more commonly diagnosed in children when they, quite noticeably, stop growing at the expected rate. It frequently happens in adults, as well. However, the symptoms are often ascribed to various other potential causes.

It's often triggered by damage to the pituitary gland, hypothalamus, or the receptors involved in regulated growth hormone.

Balance Growth Hormone with Food

We haven't yet talked about pH balance in your body, but it's another very important predictor of overall health.

Your neural, or balanced, pH is 7. Anything less than that is considered alkaline, and if it is higher than that, it's acidic.

The Standard American Diet (SAD) sabotages pH levels. Coffee, dairy, animal products, sugar, simple carbs, and fried foods all tilt the scale toward acidity and are consumed regularly by Americans. On the other hand, leafy greens and vegetables, which are consumed in my lower proportion, the trend toward alkaline.

The growth hormone is influenced by pH levels in your blood, being suppressed when you're acidic, and flourishing in an alkaline environment (Schwalfenberg, 2011).

As we discussed in the previous chapter, thyroid hormone is critical in the production of growth hormone, so anything that disrupts your thyroid function, particularly food intolerances and autoimmune disorders, will also affect your growth hormone production.

What to Eliminate and Avoid

Gluten has been the most inflammatory item removed from your diet so far, but for the next three days specifically, and preferably for the remainder of the reset, you're going to remove dairy.

The vast majority of food intolerances come from one of these two substances, and removing them from your diet for a short period of time will help your gut heal, whether or not you are personally sensitive to them.

Dairy is well known to be a significant cause of inflammation in your body. A healthy immune system responds to injury and sickness by protecting the damaged area with inflammation. Unfortunately, chronic inflammation is thought to be the root cause of almost all preventable diseases and is most certainly a contributing factor to weight gain and resistance to weight loss.

By removing dairy from your eating plan, you're highly likely to notice a reduction in symptoms like fatigue, IBS, anxiety, and fluid retention or bloating.

Approximately 75% of people around the world have difficulty processing lactose, the carbohydrate found in dairy. Percentages increase for those of African American, Asian, Native American, or Mexican American descent, and also for anyone with gluten sensitivity.

As you age, your body stops being able to produce the enzyme lactase, which is needed to break down the lactose in dairy. This results in highly uncomfortable digestive distress, leading to bloating and gas, diarrhea, and/or gastroesophageal reflux (GERD), which you'll feel in the form of heartburn.

Dairy is a major trigger for dysregulated gut health, specifically the proteins casein and whey.

Casein is a protein in milk that your immune system frequently mistakes for an intruder, creating an aggressive immune response against it, usually representing like allergies: skin reactions, sneezing, itchy eyes, possible swelling of lips, tongue, mouth or throat and, in severe cases, anaphylaxis

Whey is a different protein that will cause a similar, though unrelated, immune response. Whey can be harder to avoid because it's commonly used in protein supplements and food products, so read labels carefully!

Women have a more sensitive immune response than men, which is great in a healthy body, but if your microbiome is damaged or your hormones are unbalanced, it puts you at a much higher chance of developing an autoimmune disorder.

What to Enjoy More of

By removing dairy from your diet, you'll also be removing key nutrients that are either naturally occurring in milk products or added to them. As such, you'll want to focus on integrating high-quality alternative sources of calcium, potassium, and vitamin D.

For calcium, you can increase your intake of:

- chia seeds are a great source of dairy-free calcium because they're also high in boron, which helps your body actually to metabolize the calcium effectively

- almonds, sunflower seeds, and sesame seeds have high levels of calcium as well as healthy fats

- tofu, white beans, and edamame are not only excellent sources of dairy-free calcium, but they're all high in clean protein as well

- for vegetables, consider adding broccoli rabe, kale, sweet potato, collard greens, arugula, and butternut squash to your menu

Most fruits and vegetables are rich in potassium, so as long as your eating plenty of plant-based foods, you shouldn't need to worry about this mineral.

Dairy-free sources of Vitamin D:

- most milk alternatives will be fortified with vitamin D, just like dairy is, so make the simple swap to organic soy, almond, coconut, or hemp milk

- Fish, particularly salmon, mackerel and trout are also high in Vitamin D

- Egg yolks are also great sources of vitamin D, just make sure you are opting for pasture-raised, organic eggs for quality

Additional Tips for Naturally Regulating Growth Hormone

Removing dairy from your eating plan might be a bit of a painful process, but the more you know about what you're eating, the more determined you'll be to clean up your dietary habits.

To help stimulate healthy production of growth hormone, you can also subject your body to some healthy stressors as opposed to the negative, damaging stress that causes dysregulation.

How you move your body and how often you exercise can have a big impact on the proper regulation of growth hormone in your body. If you want to tap into this "fountain of youth," you'll have to pay just as much attention to your exercise routine as your eating patterns.

Exercise

One of the most effective ways to increase growth hormone through physical exercise is to practice High-Intensity Interval Training (HIIT) or burst exercise a few times a week.

Generally, it involves sprinting of sorts. For a short burst, usually around 20 - 30 seconds, you push your body to about 80% of your maximum heart rate, and when you return to a few minutes of low-intensity movement. You would repeat this 4 - 5 times over a 20 -30 minutes exercise session.

By incorporating high-intensity bursts, you increase your VO2 max, which is the amount of oxygen you're consuming.

In regular aerobic exercise, your body will take in more oxygen to fuel the workout. Oxygen alone isn't enough to support the anaerobic bursts involved in HIIT, so your body starts to burn fat to keep up with the demand of your workout.

To do this, your body needs to increase the amount of growth hormone circulating in your blood.

Adding sprints to your exercise routine will also lower insulin levels by burning excess blood sugar.

Avoiding Conventional Animal Products

Hormones are regularly pumped into animals to fatten them up so that farms and farmers can make more money per animal. When you eat that meat, you're ingesting those hormones too... and they'll fatten you up as well.

This is especially true in the dairy industry, where the cows are injected with a variety of hormones that help them continue to produce great quantities of milk.

Anyone alive today is likely familiar with the saying, "does a body good," in reference to milk. It turns out this might be more of a marketing ploy than actual truth.

We've been raised to consider milk as a critical source of calcium, potassium, and vitamin D, believing it to be crucial to the development and maintenance of healthy bones.

There is actually very little reliable scientific backing for milk, and most of what's available can be associated with—in other words, paid for by the dairy industry, which makes it suspect at best. As we've already pointed out, there are plenty of non-dairy sources of healthy calcium that don't cause allergic reactions in 75% of people.

Dairy is also highly addictive. Casomorphins are opioids found in dairy that have powerfully addictive qualities. In a way, this is nature's foolproof method to make sure babies drink milk to grow.

But nature will eventually reduce milk supply, encouraging the weaning process. A healthy baby will only eat when hungry, so when solid foods start being introduced, they'll naturally drink less breast milk, gradually weaning them off without causing severe symptoms of withdrawal.

When adults consume dairy regularly, and in high quantities, they become addicted.

Moreover, the hormones in milk concentrate in fat, which is why many people have a harder time giving up cheese, which has a high-fat content than skim milk, for example.

You may experience withdrawal symptoms when you eliminate dairy, but once you've broken your addiction, it will lose much of its appeal, making it easier to say "no" to dairy the longer you abstain from it.

Chapter 9:

Testosterone

Just as women naturally produce more estrogen hormones, men naturally produce more testosterone hormones. Testosterone boosts metabolism and helps the owners of said hormone stay lean, more easily burning fat and building muscle mass. In a world where excess weight is not overly desirable, this may strike a lot of women as "unfair."

Similar to progesterone production, as women age–especially after 35–testosterone production decreases steadily. Testosterone production goes down with each of these conditions:

- Post-menopause

- ovary removal or decrease of ovarian function caused by chemotherapy

- Pituitary or adrenal gland dysfunction

In men, the production of testosterone is one of the primary concerns of the testes. Women obviously don't have testes, but the small amount of testosterone they do produce is divided between their ovaries and adrenal glands.

Many of the suggestions made in the first reset that encouraged the lowering of estrogen will have a similar balancing effect on testosterone. You've been working on this hormone right from the start!

Testosterone Effects

Testosterone is a sex hormone, so its primary purpose is dedicated to increasing reproductive and sexual function. Having too much or too little of this hormone can result in a loss of libido, but having too little can also cause fertility issues.

The hormone is also designed to help your body build muscle and burn body fat, as well as enhance mood. Imbalances in this hormone, even though women require very little of it, can have significant side effects.

Low testosterone is more common because it has an inverse relationship to estrogen. When estrogen is high, testosterone dips low and vice versa. Some consequences of low testosterone include:

- increase in signs of aging, such as wrinkles, rapid muscle loss, which is undesirable on its own, but also leads to saggy skin and bone density issues like osteopenia or osteoporosis

- symptoms of menopause, such as hot flashes, irritability, mood swings, and reproductive challenges

- low sex drive, weakness, fatigue, thinning hair

In extreme cases, low testosterone has even been linked to cardiovascular disease and cancer.

High testosterone, on the other hand, is less common but has equally severe consequences.

- an increase in masculine traits, such as abnormal body hair growth, male pattern baldness, deepening voice, shrinking breasts, and irregular menstrual cycles

- increased body fat, especially around the midsection

A little goes a long when it comes to testosterone in a woman's body, and an imbalance can be dangerous.

Causes of Unbalanced Testosterone

Endocrine disruptors, particularly found in birth control and environmental toxins, are confusing our body's natural communication system, making it nearly impossible to *naturally* produce the correct amount of sex hormone for optimal health.

Damage or disruption to glands that produce complementary hormones, such as your adrenals, thyroid, and pituitary, can also cause an imbalance of your testosterone production, either high or low, depending on the relationship with the triggering hormones.

Low testosterone in women is becoming endemic, at least in part due to the prevalence of other imbalanced hormones, particularly estrogen.

Raised levels of cortisol, as you know, cause you to gain and store fat, especially around the midsection. It also contributes to poor sleep quality and dysregulated blood sugar. The cortisol spike itself, as well as the results of high cortisol, all act against the natural production of testosterone.

Low-fat diets, as well as statin drugs that are made to lower cholesterol, can also cause low testosterone.

High testosterone in women is most commonly caused by taking exogenous testosterone supplements, adrenal disorders, and a condition called PCOS, or polycystic ovarian syndrome.

PCOS doesn't currently have a definitive known cause, but it is thought to be related to metabolic disorders and high insulin.

Balance Testosterone with Food

It's clear that the human body is designed to cope with stress and toxins, but not at the level we're currently exposing ourselves to. When it comes to balancing your testosterone levels with food, it is more important that you pay attention to the production and storage than the food itself.

We're exposed to hundreds, if not thousands of toxins every day, from the cosmetics and beauty products we put on our skin and hair, to the cleaners and household items we handle. Even the air we breathe and the water we drink contain toxins and heavy metals that can damage our endocrine system.

While we can't eliminate them all, we can try not to ingest them on purpose.

Unless it's certified organic, environmental toxins in our food include:

- pesticides and herbicides

- fertilizers

- synthetic hormones

Looking at the materials, your food is packaged and stored in is also important, as aluminum cans and plastic are known to be very damaging to your health.

What to Eliminate and Avoid

Endocrine disruptors, and particularly estrogen disruptors, are found in the chemicals that are used to grow your food and the plastics you store your food in. In order to avoid adding more to the already overwhelmed state of your body, you'll have to change a few shopping habits.

You've probably heard of BPA, or bisphenol A. It's a chemical used to make plastics and resins and rose in infamy over the past few years for being associated with infertility and a host of other health disorders.

You may or may not be familiar with the consequences, but you've no doubt seen plenty of products claiming to be "BPA free." This alone creates the impression that you want to avoid it. The problem is that, while BPA might be on everyone's radar, BPF and BPS and other BPA substitutes that have nearly the same chemical makeup are being used instead.

Calling attention to one toxin to hide the presence of another is a very effective marketing technique. Just because you choose water bottles and Tupperware containers that are BPA free does not mean they are safe for your health (Gregor, M., 2017).

When you store your food or buy packaged food items, which are hopefully becoming less common on your grocery lists, prioritize glass or stainless steel containers that won't leach harmful chemicals in your food.

Liquids can be particularly susceptible, so be highly conscious of your beverage choices.

If you must use plastic containers, keep them away from heat at all times. Don't heat up your food in plastic, put food into plastic containers while it's still hot, or even leave it exposed to sunlight. Plastic has been shown to leach chemicals out of plastic and into your food by 55 faster when it's heated (Biello, 2008).

What to Enjoy More of

First and foremost, you want to do everything you can to support your liver, your body's primary detoxifying organ. Choosing foods based on specific minerals and nutrients is a good start, but you also want to make sure you aren't adding more toxins to your body in the process.

Now more than ever, it's important that you buy organic produce whenever possible. The chemicals and pesticides used on conventional crops are highly disruptive to your body's natural production of estrogen, which, in turn, dysregulates testosterone production.

Some of the most beneficial minerals for your liver are:

- Magnesium, best consumed in leafy greens, nuts and seeds, legumes, and cold-water fish such as salmon, mackerel and tuna

- Sulfur, which can be found in coconut and olive oils, radishes, watercress, arugula, kale, broccoli, Brussels sprouts, blue-green algae, spirulina, hemp, pumpkin seeds

- Selenium has the highest concentration in Brazil nuts

- Zinc and Copper are often found in the same foods, particularly in shellfish like oysters and lobster, an alga called spirulina, nuts, seeds, and legumes

One further food item that you might want to consider to support your liver is, in fact, liver. It is considered a superfood by many because it's packed with healthy protein, vitamins, and minerals are crucial to your survival.

If you enjoy the liver, make sure you are eating a healthy liver. Always choose organic, hormone-free, pasture-raised organ meat and ethics allowing, the younger liver, the better, so calf or lamb liver can be especially potent.

Bone broth is also a helpful way to help your liver remove toxins from your body, and it helps in the repair process as well. There are amino acids in bone broth that stimulate collagen production, encouraging a healthy inflammation response in your body as well as tightening and toning your skin.

Finally, you want to make sure you're drinking plenty of clean, filtered water. This is not the same as bottled water, which not only comes in plastic, but it often is no different than the water from your tap. Getting a simple, activated carbon or charcoal water filter for your fridge at home is an inexpensive way to help you drink more healthy, clean water to support your body's natural detoxification process.

Additional Tips for Supporting Testosterone Levels

Testosterone production is one of your hormones that is heavily influenced by the environment you are situated in, every day. Yes, of course, stress is a large factor, but how you move your body and what types and varieties of external toxins you're exposed to play a critical role as well.

Sex hormones are one of the easiest for medical science to synthetically duplicate, which is why women are often prescribed birth control to deal with excess estrogen-related issues. Synthetic testosterone is also frequently prescribed, as is medication designed to block testosterone receptors, depending on whether your body is producing too much or too little of the hormone.

But just because we *can* trick our body into thinking everything is rebalanced, doesn't mean we necessarily *should*.

Exercise

Naturally stimulating your endocrine system to produce, use, and eliminate testosterone as your body actually requires is the best solution to hormone management. One of the simplest ways to do this is to exercise.

Yoga helps to realign your entire body, inside and out, improving digestion and natural detoxification. It also improves breathing, and oxygen is a powerful natural detoxification tool.

Resistance or weight training to build muscle stimulates growth hormone and testosterone production. A lot of women get nervous at the idea of weight training because they don't want to end up looking bulky and masculine. This is not a very substantial risk, however, because even men have to work really hard to get bulky themselves, and they naturally produce a lot more testosterone. It's rare for women to get bulky and only happens with specific training measures and supplementation.

Balancing your hormones isn't about producing a lot of testosterone; it's about producing the right amount of testosterone for health.

Interval training, using sprints, bursts, or HIIT has also been shown to increase the production of both growth hormone and testosterone, and as an added bonus, this method of training is the least time consuming to see results.

Supplements vs. Medications

There are plenty of frequently prescribed medications and bioidentical hormones that can synthetically "balance" your hormones. What they really do is drive your levels beyond their normal range, regardless of how your biological system responds to them. In other words, there is no "off" button to medications.

There are a place and time for everything, but if you're using medicine or bioidentical hormones, you have to monitor all your hormone levels carefully and often. They may also have a negative effect on HDL, so it's a good idea to monitor cholesterol as well.

Generalizing the situation, medications suppress and hide symptoms, whereas holistic measures help address the root cause to heal the problem.

Diet and lifestyle changes aren't introducing hormones to your body; they're stimulating the natural production of hormones for optimal, balanced biological processes to occur.

In addition to the changes already encouraged, you can also look into a family of herbs called "adaptogens." These are plants that help your body adapt to and deal with stressors. They were mentioned briefly in Chapter 6 as a way to manage cortisol levels, and that practice can also help balance your testosterone.

Ashwagandha, for example, has been shown to decrease cortisol, increase DHEA, and thereby increase free testosterone levels. Look for a root extract that includes 'withanolides."

Toxins and Heavy Metals

Understanding the dangers of toxins and heavy metals are important, but it might also help to understand how they are stored and released into your body.

All hormones interact with cells using receptors that are either inside the cell, for fat-soluble hormones, or along the outer cell wall, in the case of water-soluble hormones.

Toxins and heavy metals are often stored in adipose or fat tissues and are difficult to get rid of because your body is protecting itself from the toxins by hiding them away in your fat cells where they can't do much damage.

Sex hormones are all fat-soluble, so while these toxins are hiding out in your fat cells, they disrupt your hormone receptors for estrogen, progesterone, testosterone, cortisol, and thyroid hormone. You may have noticed that these hormones interact very closely with each other.

Metals that are known to accumulate in your body include:

- mercury, cadmium, lead, and arsenic

Some level of heavy metals is expected, and your body can handle. Unfortunately, overexposure has made toxicity a problem.

There are many ways humans are exposed to heavy metals and other endocrine-disrupting chemicals, such as:

- ○ passed on through pregnancy/birth

- ○ environmental factors: toys, paint, household items

- ○ work: construction industry, salons, printing industry

- ○ dental work: metals and/or mercury in fillings

- ○ antiperspirants and aluminum foil

- ○ vaccines: particularly in the past, mercury compounds were used in vaccines as a preservative

- ○ processed foods and natural foods: these metals are in the soil, which means they're in the plants and everything that eats plants

○ cosmetics and hygiene products: especially look out for parabens, phthalates, sodium lauryl sulfate, each of which is well-known estrogen-mimicking chemicals

Toxicity has been linked to serious diseases and disorders:

○ autism, ADD, ADHD are linked to heavy metal toxicity

○ cancer

○ imbalanced immune system

○ syndromes such as IBS and fibromyalgia

○ neurodegenerative diseases like Alzheimer's, Parkinson's and Dementia

Everything you're doing to heal your natural testosterone balance can also help remove toxins from your body. When you detox a lot of toxins rapidly, as happens when you lose a lot of weight quickly or suddenly integrate detoxing agents into your eating plan, you might not be able to eliminate them quickly enough, and your body will start to reabsorb them, fitting them back into your fat cells.

If this happens on mass, you may experience symptoms like gas, bloating, skin rash, loose bowels, or nausea. In other words, you may feel worse before you feel better.

Chapter 10:

What to do after Your Reset

The last thing you want to do after going through the commitment of the past 21 days is to return to old habits that will throw your hormones right back out of sync. You don't have to be on a diet for the rest of your life, but you should establish new patterns of eating that will support your hormones and your overall health.

Now that your hormones are back in balance, it'll be much easier to understand the cues your body is giving you. Without the confusion and mixed messages of a broken metabolism, your body should be telling you the truth more often than not now.

It's your job to learn to listen to your body and understand what it's telling you, instead of selectively intuiting only what you want to hear. When you give your body a chance to heal, you might be surprised at how often you crave "healthy" foods instead of items that never fail to make you feel guilty.

Gradually Reintegrate Food

As you finalize your hormone reset, you can start to reintroduce eliminated foods back into your meal planning.

Try not to rush this process, but do so gradually by consuming them one at a time, once per day, for at least a couple of days before moving onto another reintroduction. By adding foods back one at a time, you'll not only give your gut time to readapt to the food, but you'll also know instantly if that food causes any problems for you. Your metabolism and digestive system will react instantly to any irritants, and it will be obvious what is causing the sensitivity.

Listen to your gut. If bloating, heartburn, or either constipation or diarrhea are a reaction to a change in your eating habits, don't ignore these signs. It's far better to live healthfully for the rest of your life without a particular food than to damage your body and live in pain and discomfort for the rest of your life.

Practice Mindful Eating

Before you reintroduce something that you haven't had in the past 21 days, ask yourself why you're adding it back into your eating plan. Is it to work your way back to a healthy, balanced, and sustainable eating plan? If yes, go for it, but start with small portion sizes to let your body adjust, and take notes about how your body reacts.

If you're reintroducing something that instantly makes you feel guilty, reconsider. You've just treated your body like a goddess for 21 days, do you really want to slide back into bad habits? You've come this far, if you don't want to have to detox and go through withdrawal again in six months, maybe you should just keep certain destructive foods out of your life for good. It will never be easier than now when you're healthier than you've probably been in years, and you've already kicked symptoms of withdrawal.

Practicing mindful eating can help you listen to your body's signals. Start paying close attention to *why* you're eating, whether you're actually hungry, or if you're trying to fill some other need. If you're eating for a non-hunger related issue, find something else to fill that void.

If you think you're hungry, but it's not a proper mealtime, drink a glass of water and spend five minutes doing something else to occupy your mind. If you're still hungry, have a healthy snack, like a handful of nuts. If your hunger is gone, or if you forget that you were hungry, don't eat!

If you have a craving for something specific that isn't on your ", feel great" foods list, reference the swaps list you created at the beginning of a plan. If you're hungry for something sweet, but a banana doesn't appeal to you, you're probably not hungry. Maybe you're bored, emotional, or procrastinating, and there's a better way to handle the issue.

Do you remember the days before the hormone reset when you would grab yourself a snack at night and then sit down in front of the television to enjoy your favorite show? We've all done that. No matter how determined you are to just have a few bites of this ice cream or only a handful of those chips, half an hour goes by, and we look down to find the entire pint demolished or bag emptied. Not only did you just consume a load of empty calories, but you weren't even really present enough to enjoy them!

Mindful eating is about focusing on each bite, savoring and appreciating the food you're eating, and removing distractions that lead to overeating and binge eating.

Think about actually chewing your food while you eat. The more you chew, the better you'll digest it. Also, the more in tune you are with the process of eating, the less likely you are to overeat accidentally.

Mindful eating can help you better appreciate, taste, and cherish your food.

Intermittent Fasting (IF)

Each of the hormonal imbalances we addressed over the past 21 days, particularly insulin, leptin, and cortisol, influence and are influenced by your appetite and eating patterns.

Intermittent fasting allows you to adequately rest your body, allowing it the time it needs to heal. By depleting your reserves of energy, you'll reset your entire body to function more like it did before weight was ever a problem for you.

IF has been proven to help fat burning and sustained weight loss without restricting or even counting calories.

Adjust For Sensitivities and Intolerances

As mentioned a few times already in this chapter, it's important for your long-term health that you adjust your eating plan moving forward to completely eliminate any foods that might trigger a hormonal or autoimmune response.

Having eliminated many common sensitivities for days, if not weeks, puts you in a perfect situation to notice exactly what might be bothering you, without wondering which of the ten items you ate for dinner triggered your heartburn today.

This is a good point to enlist the help of your doctor or a nutritionist, registered dietician or naturopathic professional, if you haven't already. They can perform simple sensitivity tests that should provide you with clear results now that your body has done some healing and is thinking more clearly.

Moving forward, your focus when you eat should always be to integrate as many clean, nutrient-dense foods as possible and eliminate as many empty calories and chemical/additive-laden foods as you can.

Eliminate for life:

There are some foods, beverages, and food-like items that should simply never have a place on your plate.

Conventionally produced meat and dairy are loaded with hormones and antibiotics which destroy your hormone balance and the gut microbiome.

In 2014, more than 20 million pounds of antibiotics were sold for use in animal agriculture, which represents around 80% of the total antibiotics sold during that year (Foodprint.org, 2019).

Antibiotics have saved millions of lives, and they are an incredible advancement of modern medicine, but there is no denying the fact that they also interfere with gut health and hormone balance.

If you are prescribed antibiotics to heal from a disease or injury, they might be critical to your survival. However, if you're eating them without even knowing they're in your food, they are damaging your long-term health, rather than helping it. 80% of antibiotics being pumped into conventionally farmed meat puts your health at risk.

That doesn't even take into consideration the steroid hormones being injected into livestock to make them grow big and fatty. Those hormones will also make you grow big and fatty.

Even without antibiotics and hormones to consider, industrially produced animal agriculture is typically grain-fed. These animals are lower in nutrition because they're not getting the natural vitamins (A, B, C & E) or fatty acids (omega 3s) that grass-fed animals ingest normally.

Moving forward, conventionally produced meat and dairy should not be on your grocery list, and neither should any processed meats that are filled with preservatives and additives.

There are also some oils and fats that you're going to want to avoid permanently. Healthy, natural fats are great for your body and metabolism. Highly processed oils like vegetable oils–canola, soy, corn–and anything that says partially hydrogenated are not and should be avoided at all costs.

Finally, for your long-term health, look to the beverages that you're consuming. What you drink can be one of the quickest ways to influence your hormones, particularly insulin. Stay far away from soda, commercial fruit juice, and energy drinks.

Some alcohol, coffee, and tea can be a good source of antioxidants, but their benefits are easily overcome by the detrimental burdens on your liver if you over-consume. Limit your intake, and try not to binge drink any of these beverages.

Finally, drink plenty of water, but keep it out of plastic bottles. Use stainless steel or glass bottles instead.

Enjoy for life

First, a little clarification. The last section was not meant to imply that you should never eat meat again. Instead, simply focus on organic, pasture-raised meat and dairy and eat it in moderation. Wild game can also be a tasty and healthy addition to your meal plan.

To supplement your meat, continue to eat cold-water fish that are low in mercury, like wild-caught salmon, cod, trout, sardines, anchovies. Shellfish also has many health benefits, so work crab, clams, oysters, and scallops into your cooking at least occasionally.

Finally, don't forget or forego your plant-based proteins. Legumes, certain nuts and seeds, some whole grains, and organic soy products have dense nutritional profiles that will not only supplement your clean protein intake but also provide you with a healthy collection of additional vitamins and minerals.

Many of your healthiest fats will also be in your proteins, in the animal and seafood products you eat. Nuts, seeds, and avocados are fantastic plant-based sources of nutrient-dense, healthy fat, as are certain oils. Olive, avocado, and coconut oils are high in healthy mono and polyunsaturated fats, as is organic, pasture-raised ghee.

Fruits, especially berries, lemons, and limes, can be eaten in moderation for the rest of your life unless you have a sensitivity to them or some other metabolic disorder. They are high in nutrients and fiber and a great alternative to sweets, but they are still high in sugar, so eating too many fruits can disrupt insulin and other hormones again.

Vegetables can more or less exist in unlimited quantities in the future. As long as your unique and individual biological system doesn't have a sensitivity to a particular vegetable, eat them at will and in as much variety as you can manage.

Similarly, the sky's the limit in regard to plant-based herbs and spices. Go straight to the source and avoid packaged spice combinations that are extraordinarily high in salt and potentially have chemicals and other additives like MSG.

When you're thirsty, reach for filtered water first. Consider keeping cold, naturally flavored water in your fridge so that it's available whenever you need it. You can also slowly reintroduce tea and coffee in moderation, but drink them both without sugar or dairy if possible. Kefir and kombucha are healthy, probiotic drinks that will add plenty of variety to your life if you need something a little different.

With a well-balanced eating plan, you should get most of the nutrition you need to stay healthy long-term. Due to seasonal availability of food and soil depletion, you might want to consider the option of a high-quality multivitamin, though it's a good idea to talk to your doctor or a nutritionist to decide what's best for you.

Focus on Quality

There's no need to obsess over your food or eliminate everything that could be even remotely harmful from your life forever. Instead of creating stress and anxiety around your food, begin thinking more about quality, and the rest will take care of itself.

Portion Control

As much as this entire book focused on *what* you decide to eat instead of how much you eat, quantity does still matter, if only in regard to your budget.

One of the main arguments against buying organic food is the price tag associated with it. When you set your sights on quality, you have the ability to eat less and enjoy your food and your health more.

High-quality food is more nutrient-dense, which not only means more vitamins and minerals working to keep you healthy, but it also means that each calorie you consume actually makes you feel full.

Empty calories aren't just devoid of nutrition; they're devoid of satiation. In order to fill up, you need to eat more, and more and then some more. While you're trying to fuel your body, you're creating the very hormonal imbalances that brought you to this book in the first place.

You don't have to diet for the rest of your life to maintain a healthy weight and feel great. But you do have to eat with your health in mind.

The nutritional value of organic food is much higher than industrially produced foods, and it doesn't come with the toxins, chemicals, and heavy metals that add insult to injury.

If you return to eating like you used to, you will have taken one very smart step forward only to follow it with hundreds of forkful sized steps backward.

When it comes to price, the major player is organic, hormone-free, pasture-raised meat, and dairy. If you're still concerned about the price, consider eating meat not just in smaller portions, but less frequently in your meals.

You just went 21 days without it; there's no reason you can go a few days a week without out for the rest of your life. Supplementing with high-quality organic legumes, pulses, soy, and certain grains and seeds can drastically cut the overall price of protein in your grocery bill.

At the same time, you'll be adding variety to your meals that will not just be exciting and delicious, but give you a more inclusive nutrient profile as well.

Finally, the more you–and everyone else in the world–buys organic, pasture-raised meat and dairy, the more the food industry will take notice. It's called voting with your wallet, and it works. The government currently subsidizes factory farms, but if demand shifts, so will their subsidies.

Go ahead and share this book with all your friends and family members. Hopefully, you'll be helping to improve their health as well as lower the costs of high-quality food in the long term.

The same is true for organic produce. Supply will follow demand, so choose organic at every opportunity and say no to the pollutants that are killing not just your body, but the entire world as well.

Invest in Your Health

It's not just the food that you're eating that you need to improve, but also the environment that you're living in. Everything from the air you breathe, to the water you drink and the products you put on your skin, has an impact on your health.

We've discussed environmental toxins in plastics and heavy metals. Invest in your health by buying long-lasting, high-quality food storage containers made out of glass or stainless steel. Avoid "non-stick" pans that leave slivers of chemical-laden materials in your food and invest in great stainless steel or cast iron pan. Products like this will cost more upfront, but they will last longer and be safer for you. In the long-term, it's an investment that makes sense.

You can also consider investing in a professional water filtration system for your home. Again, it comes with an upfront cost, but it will save you over time from buying either bottled water, which may not be any better for your health after all or disposable filters.

By filtering the water for your entire home, you're also protecting yourself from the chemicals and toxins in the water that you cook with and shower in.

Your skin absorbs everything it comes into contact with, including the water you wash with and the products you use to clean yourself with. Invest in your beauty products just like you invest in your food. Everything you put on your skin makes its way into your bloodstream just as surely as if you put it in your mouth and swallowed.

Take the mindset of "quality over quantity" into your life at large and let it rule your shopping habits from here on out. You and your health are worth investing in.

Chapter 11:

Physical Fitness is Always Helpful

Weight gain and retention is certainly not just about eating less and exercising more, contrary to popular opinion. But that doesn't mean physical activity isn't absolutely essential to your health.

You've heard the saying, "use it or lose it," and that couldn't be truer when it comes to your muscles and bones. Your muscles aren't just vanity features. Everything in your body operates because of muscle activity, and if you aren't moving your body on a regular basis, there will come a time when you won't be able to move your body at all.

If you're new to exercise, or if you're trying a new activity, working with a fitness professional who has a background in women's health and/or nutrition, health, and hormones can be a huge benefit.

Fitness During the 21-Day Diet

After reading this far into the book, you should be convinced that weight loss is not always about calories in versus calories out. Sometimes, your hormones make all the difference to your efforts.

When your metabolism is dysregulated and slow, exercise doesn't play as big of a role in weight loss as it would in a well-balanced body. *What* you fuel your body with is mainly responsible for weight loss success, or failure, but exercise does still make a difference.

Moving your body plays a role in balancing your hormones, so physical movement should be a part of your program right from the start. The type and intensity of activities you commit to will progress as you move forward in the reset.

Start Slow

Unless you're already an athlete, you should start slow. For the first few days, or even the first week, make it your goal to sit less simply—at least 90 minutes less if possible.

Ninety minutes add up quickly when you break up down into smaller stints. In an eight-hour workday, if you get up to walk around for five minutes every hour, you'll already have accounted for 40 minutes.

Depending on your own unique circumstance, you might consider using a standing desk, pacing around your office while you're on the phone, or simply drinking lots of water to give you a great excuse to have to walk to the bathroom every hour.

Since you'll be cooking more often, keep in mind that time spent chopping vegetables and sauteing fish is more physically taxing that time spent driving to a restaurant or ordering food from your computer.

If you've gone through your entire day and realize you didn't have a chance to move your body at all, instead of sitting down to watch an hour of television after dinner, cut it back to half an hour and spend the other time strolling around the block with your significant other, pet, or just your inner self.

It is a good idea to choose a time of day when you will be able to dedicate 20 - 30 minutes to exercise in the long term. You don't have to start out by training for a marathon or weight lifting competition, but simply getting used to a set time of day that is dedicated to movement is a good habit-forming base that will be helpful when you're ready to step up the intensity.

Increase Intensity

During the Insulin Reset, it can really help to burn off some glucose daily. Adding a short interval or burst into your current routine can be a great opportunity to get you accustomed to stepping up the intensity without adding a lot of stress to your workout commitment.

For example, if you've been going for an after-dinner walk for 30 minutes each evening, add a few sprints. Walk leisurely for five minutes, jog for 30 seconds, walk briskly for five more minutes, run for 30 seconds, walk briskly for five more minutes, sprint for 30 seconds, etc. This is a slow introduction to interval training that has been shown to improve insulin sensitivity and raise growth hormone greatly.

By the time you've successfully hit the leptin reset, your metabolism will be ready to start putting exercise to proper use in your weight loss efforts. When you first start to increase the intensity, focus on healing your body through stress-relieving activities, and realignment focused movements.

Start by being more intentional about your physical movements. Speed walking, hiking, or jogging out in nature are great stress relievers and easy ways to build up your endurance safely. You can also try swimming or bike riding.

Movements that realign your skeletal and modulatory body will also help realign your organs and digestive system, making your internal processes more effective. Practices such as yoga, Pilates, or barre class are great ways to step up the intensity of your fitness efforts in a safe, controlled, and restorative manner.

Above all, be safe. Work with a personal trainer if you're new to fitness, at least to get you started so that a) you'll be monitored and b) you'll learn the correct postures, positions, and movements, so you don't accidentally hurt yourself.

Fitness after the 21-Day Diet

Once your hormones are reset, you'll be ready to start focusing on other areas of health in your life, including your fitness. The reset focused primarily on your diet because the research shows that weight loss is primarily determined by what you put on your fork.

Making sure the weight stays gone, however, can be heavily influenced by your physical activity levels.

Exercise is an important component not just in your future hormone health, but in helping you stay youthful, strong, and energetic no matter what your age.

Depending on where your fitness levels are right now, you'll want to continue adjusting the intensity of your fitness upward as you get stronger and more fit. When it comes to exercise, it's always better to play it safe and work your way up gradually.

There are two forms of exercise that have been shown to improve hormonal health, and they also have anti-aging results: High-Intensity Interval Training (HIIT) and resistance or weight training.

Interval Training and Yoga

For many years, we've been told that if you want to lose weight, you have to do cardio. Lots of cardio. Science, not to mention millions of women worldwide who continue to lose weight on the treadmill, is finally telling a different story.

High-Intensity Interval Training (HIIT) is ideal in so many ways. First of all, it allows you to get an entire workout completed in only 20 - 30 minutes. It boosts the production of human growth hormone, which helps to stimulate fat loss and lean muscle production, and it doesn't overstress your body like endurance training can, causing a spike in your cortisol levels.

HIIT is simple and variable. You can apply it to nearly any type of exercise you enjoy the most, whether that's jogging, riding your bike, swimming or dancing. The goal is simple: add 30-second sprints of high intensity that push you past your comfort zone and require about 80% of your maximum heart rate.

Follow the sprints with a recovery period of around 40% of your maximum heart rate for 10 seconds and repeat the process three times for a total of three minutes. Once you've done one set, rest for two minutes, and then switch up the intervals for another three minutes session. Do this five times, and you've accomplished a very effective workout in only 25 minutes.

You only need to do this 25-minute work out three times a week to see better results that you experience running for hours a week on a treadmill.

To give your body the best stress-reducing recovery possible, you can incorporate yoga into your HIIT practice. Yoga is known as a relaxing, somewhat meditative activity that is wonderful for aligning your body and increasing zen. This is all true and very beneficial, but yoga and also work up a good sweat and create some beautiful, lean muscles.

To work it into your HIIT routine, do 30-second bursts of high-intensity bodyweight movements in between your yoga poses. Some great examples are mountain climbers, burpees, high knee sprints, jumping ropes, or ice skaters.

Resistance or Weight Training

Resistance training and weight training both focus on building muscle, and both have incredible benefits for your overall health.

Muscle is built through a natural process of damage and repair. Your body has a response dedicated specifically to helping you repair microtears in your muscles so that they grow stronger over time. It is natural and healthy.

Resistance training, as you might be able to guess, uses resistance to challenge your muscles, such as body weight or rowing a boat through the water.

Weight training, on the other hand, uses either free weights or weight machines to challenge your muscles beyond their normal use. For example, doing a bicep curl with an empty hand is going to provide you with very limited muscle usage, but if you lift a five or 10-pound weight, you'll be taxing your muscles.

In terms of helping you lose weight and keep it off when you focus on weight training, you get the benefits of what's called "afterburn." Because you've created damage to your muscles and stimulated your internal repair process, your metabolism also speeds up in order to fuel this extra repair process. This boost to your metabolism can burn additional energy for anywhere between 4 - 8 hours.

Building muscles puts stress on your muscles, but not necessarily on the rest of your body. This means you can enjoy the positive effects of a great workout without the downsides of increasing cortisol, provided you don't overextend your limits.

This is great news for women because it means not only do you never have to worry about bulking up, but you also can stick to shorter workouts, saving you time.

For best fitness results after your hormone reset, work your way up to three 20 - 30 minute HIIT workouts a week, incorporating yoga if you can, and two 30 minute resistance or weight training workouts.

Remember to enlist the services of a professional whenever you're learning new movements or routines. There are no benefits to hurting yourself while trying to improve your health.

Find the Right Fitness for You

How you exercise when you're 20 probably looks a lot different from how you will exercise when your 50 or even 80 years old. And it should.

At different stages of your life, your body needs different kinds of support.

When you're young and nimble, you can challenge your body in unique ways with less risk of injury. This is a great time to experiment and see what types of activity make you feel great and keep your interest. Setting a good foundation of cardio, strength training, and flexibility work will help you move through life in good condition.

Playing against your strengths will help you keep balanced. For women, this is more likely to look like weight training, whereas men might focus more on flexibility.

When you hit your mid-30s, your metabolism shifts, and with it, so should your exercise patterns. You might have to work a little harder to keep the weight from packing on and struggle a little bit more with the recovery time.

Did someone mention time? You probably have less of it to devote to exercise at this point in your life, so resistance training and high-intensity interval training (HIIT) will give you the best results in the shortest period of time.

Both those activities will also help you be proactive about bone health and muscle loss.

As you continue to age into your 40s and 50s, your fitness focus should be on maintaining your muscle mass and protecting your bones. Strength training and resistance exercises that also incorporate mobility and flexibility movements are perfect for this age group.

Consider activities like bodyweight based interval training, hiking, and Pilates.

Fitness in your 60s and beyond will depend heavily on your condition going into them. If you're already fit, continue doing what is working for you, but move toward lower-impact activities that still protect your bones and encourage muscle retention. If you're a runner, consider spending some time in swimming pools instead as needed.

You need to pay attention to your focus, controlling your movements carefully, and ensuring you are always stable and protected.

Have Fun

Exercise shouldn't be a punishment. It should be a reward. Life is hard, and moving your body should be fun, making you feel young and energetic again. Think about the happiest kids you've ever seen. What makes them so joyful? Running around, playing sports, and having fun.

If you can find a fitness routine that you enjoy and look forward to, you'll be much more likely to find a way to work exercise into your life. If you dread the thought of having to exercise, you might just give up before you even give yourself a chance to get stronger.

If you're new to fitness, take some time to experiment with different options.

Join a gym, take some classes, hire a personal trainer for a few weeks. You may find that group activities keep you motivated and help you enjoy your workouts. Or maybe beating your personal bests in a competition against yourself is what keeps you going.

You may find that working out inside, in a structured environment, makes you feel safe and focused, or an outdoor boot camp might get your heart racing with excitement.

Don't feel like there's only one way to stay fit. There are thousands of options for you to move your body, and finding the right choice for you is an individual decision.

Don't Hurt Yourself

The absolute most important factor in fitness is not to hurt yourself. Whether you're new to fitness or you've just been given a new burst of energy thanks to the hormone reset, it's important that you start at a level that is appropriate for your current state.

Jumping in too far too fast can end up in injury, and the last thing you want is another excuse to let your health and fitness degenerate.

Working with a professional and taking your time in any new fitness routine will help ensure you're able to continue moving your body every day for the rest of your life.

Conclusion

Life is much too valuable to waste feeling tired, weak, and in pain. Your body was meant to be full of energy, vitality, and get up and go. It's time you got that feeling back and held onto it for life.

This isn't about what the number on the scale says. That's just a byproduct. The more fantastic you feel, the better that number is going to look to you.

We live in a world that puts a lot of emphasis on size, clothes, and the current standards of beauty. The problem with those standards is that it's not really the size of the clothes the women in the magazine are wearing that you envy. It's their smile.

It's the implication that the beautiful women of the world are happy that makes the rest of the women in the world want to be like them. Women of the world have been struggling for decades to look like the women on the cover of magazines, even knowing that nothing about those standards are natural or even attainable.

It's time to stop killing yourself for the byproduct of what you really want, and start working toward the real goal: health and happiness.

Eating less and exercising more isn't going to bring you joy. It's probably not even going to change the numbers on the scale very much. It will make you miserable, though, if you work at it hard enough.

There is a better way.

Instead of punishing your body for damage beyond its control, you can start to appreciate it for all the hard work it does. You can nourish it and treat it with the love and constant devotion that it deserves. That you deserve.

Resetting your hormones isn't just about helping you lose weight. It's about guiding you toward life-long health that lets you live life to the fullest, enjoying every moment along the way.

An Effective Hormone Reset Diet

The recommendations outlined in this 21-Day Hormone Reset program are designed to help you get your metabolic system back in order by supporting your hormone-producing endocrine system.

The human body is remarkable. In as little as three days, your hormones can find their way back to homeostasis, provided nothing is confusing them or getting in their way.

Modern life is just as exciting and joyful as it is stressful, and balance needs to be addressed from all angles. Every decision you make throughout the day will affect your health, and the more you can trend toward health instead of away from it, the more you'll be able to enjoy all life has to offer.

By addressing the food you eat, removing items that cause disruption, and adding items that offer nourishment, you can support the systems of your body. A well-fueled body is designed to provide constant energy, stable moods, quick thinking, and unconscious weight management.

All the really hard work is done by your hormones. Your hormones are in charge of keeping your heart beating and your digestion moving. They protect you from disease and injury and brain damage.

In return, you feed them.

If you follow a Standard American Diet full of processed food, sugar, synthetic hormones, toxins, and heavy metals, you are feeding them poison.

On the other hand, if you feed them organic, natural proteins, fats, and plenty of vitamin and mineral-packed, plant-based carbohydrates, you'll be protecting and healing them just as surely as they protect and heal you.

Everything in nature follows a cycle. You get what you put in. Your body is very forgiving, and in as little as 21 days, you can see real health results. If you treat it like a crash diet, those results will fade just as quickly as your healthy habits do.

But if you change your lifestyle to support your health, these results can last a lifetime.

Sustaining Hormone Health for Life

Dieting is a thing of a modern, media-driven world, but it can be a thing of your past. None of them have ever worked for you before, or you wouldn't have read this book.

Calorie-based diets don't work in the long-term. Exercise obsessions are impractical and dangerous and, for most women, don't work either.

If you want to see a change in your body, a change in your health, you need to change how you treat your body. The Hormone Reset Diet is only a short, 21-day commitment to getting you started.

How you feel the rest of your life will depend on how committed to the changes, you are.

Do you want to wake up every morning feeling well-rested and ready to take on the day?

Would you love to be able to go on weekend adventures with friends and family, knowing that you not only have the energy, but you also can rely on your digestion to be on its best behavior?

Do you want to go out dancing, having the time of your life and fielding pick up lines all night long because you look so damn good, everyone in the room wants to get to know you better?

When you get hungry, would you like to reach for delicious food that you know is going to give you a better jolt of energy than the best double-espresso ever did? Do you want to impress your friends and family by feeding them "healthy" food that tastes better and is more satisfying than their favorite delivery?

Life is meant to be enjoyed. It's yours for the taking.

It won't always be easy, but it can be simple. You can stop agonizing over everything that has gone wrong in the past, and start appreciating everything that is ready to go right for you in the future.

The Hormone Reset Diet is just the beginning. You have the rest of your life ahead of you to feel this great and so much better.

Take care of yourself.

References

Biello, D. (2008, February 19). Plastic (Not) Fantastic: Food Containers Leach a Potentially Harmful Chemical [Web log post]. *Scientific American.* Retrieved September 18, 2019, from https://www.scientificamerican.com/article/plastic-not-fantastic-with-bisphenol-a/

Breastcancer.org. (2019). U.S. Breast Cancer Statistics. Retrieved September 13, 2019, from https://www.breastcancer.org/symptoms/understand_bc/statistics

Circadian rhythm. (n.d.). In Wikipedia. Retrieved September 17, 2019, from https://en.wikipedia.org/wiki/Circadian_rhythm

Foodprint.org. (2019). Antibiotics in Our Food System [Web log post]. Retrieved September 18, 2019, from https://foodprint.org/issues/antibiotics-in-our-food-system/

Gottfried, S. (n.d.). 15 Reasons To Rethink Red Meat [Web log post]. Retrieved September 13, 2019, from https://www.mindbodygreen.com/0-18145/15-reasons-to-rethink-red-meat.html

Gregor, M. [NutritionFacts.org] (2017, April 12). Are the BPA-free Alternatives Safe? [Video file]. Retrieved from https://youtu.be/QuMGcoEswTc

Qualiani, D,. Felt-Gunderson, P., (2017). Closing America's Fiber Intake Gap. *American Journal of Lifestyle Medicine,* 11(1), 80-85. doi: 10.1177/1559827615588079

Schwalfenberg, G. K. (2011, August 8). The Alkaline Diet: Is There Evidence That an Alkaline pH Diet Benefits Health? *Journal of Environmental and Public Health.* 2012. 7 pages. http://dx.doi.org/10.1155/2012/727630

Stachowicz, A. & Lebiedzinska, A. (2016, December). The effect of diet components on the level of cortisol. *European Food Research and Technology.* 242(12), 2001-2009. Retrieved from https://doi.org/10.1007/s00217-016-2772-3

Vanderpump, M. P. J. (2011, September). The epidemiology of thyroid disease. *British Medical Bulletin*, 99(1). 39–51. https://doi.org/10.1093/bmb/ldr030

Waldie, Paul. (2018, April 23). Protective mother wrestles lost polar bear. *The Globe And Mail Canada.* Retrieved from https://www.theglobeandmail.com/news/national/protective-mother-wrestles-lost-polar-bear/article703773/

Wellness Resources. (2008). The Leptin Diet: The 5 Rules of the Leptin Diet [Video File]. Retrieved from https://youtu.be/NwdxTRAH_Gs

Appendix 1: Meal Planning

The meals suggested in this section are not recipes, but rather guides to help you become more familiar with the foods that this reset encourages you to eat.

There are no quantities and no specific cooking times because each meal is designed to suit your own taste preferences. You can add variety in many ways, and each slight alteration will require a slightly different cooking time.

By using high quality, nutrient-dense ingredients and eating mindfully, your body will naturally tell you when it has had enough to eat, and counting calories shouldn't be necessary if you listen to your body's signals.

Get creative with the following meal suggestions and try to change up the ingredients every time you cook each dish to take in the most nutrients and minerals.

Breakfast Scramble

Starting your day with a healthy helping of clean, lean protein will help you maintain steady energy levels throughout the day, as well as kickstart your metabolism.

Since you'll be avoiding meat for the next 21 days, this breakfast scramble will provide you with plenty of options to mix and match proteins, as well as vary the other ingredients. With a little creativity, you can have a unique breakfast every day.

Ingredients

Start with your protein. Choose one of the following to be your base:

- organic, pasture-raised eggs

- organic tofu

- organic tempeh

- lentils

- quinoa

Add your healthy fats. Choose one of the following to saute your scramble:

- Extra Virgin Olive Oil

- Avocado Oil

- Coconut Oil

- Organic Ghee

You can also add some fresh avocado once your scramble is cooked. You don't need much oil, and always keep in mind that it's highly concentrated, so a little goes a long way. Eggs and soy-based proteins also have healthy fats in them, in a nature-intended balance of protein to fat.

Finally, add your carbs in the form of vegetables.

- at least one leafy greens, such as spinach, kale, orchard

- 2 - 3 other colorful veggies, such as broccoli, bell peppers, asparagus, zucchini, mushrooms, hot peppers

Lentils and quinoa are also high in carbohydrates, but we're not trying to focus on calories or macros. We're focusing on the quality and types of ingredients, making sure that what you're taking in supports optimal hormone production and regulation.

You can also add herbs and spices to flavor your scramble. Choose from any of the following or add your own personal favorites to the list:

- onion

- garlic

- basil

- rosemary

- cayenne

Try to choose fresh herbs when possible or dried herbs if you must. Avoid anything packed in oil or combined into a preformulated mix. Check the ingredients list to make sure the only thing listed is the herb you're planning on eating.

Directions

If you're using eggs, beat them raw in a bowl first. If you're using quinoa or lentils, have it pre-cooked and cooled. For a scramble made with tofu, crumble firm or extra firm tofu directly into a pan. Tempeh won't necessarily crumble, but you can break or cut it into small chunks.

Add your protein, oils, and finely chopped onion, if you're using it, to a pan on medium heat and start to sauté your scramble.

After a few minutes, add your chopped veggies and continue to mix everything until the vegetables are nicely cooked but not too soft.

If you're using garlic or other herbs, add them last, when there are only 2 minutes left to the cooking process.

Buddha Bowls

One of the most common signs of insulin resistance is constant hunger and the feeling that you need to eat every few hours. This is not ideal for survival or your hormones, so your new eating plan goal is to provide your body with enough sustainable energy to get you through four to five hours between meals.

Eating sufficient high-quality protein and healthy fats will help. You should already be eating protein-packed breakfasts, thanks to the Estrogen Reset Breakfast Scrambles, so now it's time to focus on your lunch, which can be more difficult to work protein into without relying on processed meats.

Buddha bowls have been popularized in recent years as vegetarian and vegan lifestyles have grown in popularity, and they're a great lunch option. They can be made ahead of time, focus on high quality, clean proteins, and incorporate healthy, low glycemic carbs and delicious fats.

They're also versatile enough that you can enjoy a different bowl every day of the week to avoid boredom and expand your flavor horizon.

Ingredients

Choose one of the following to be your protein-packed base:

- quinoa

- wild or brown rice

- cooked lentils or black beans

Add an extra protein (optional & pre-cooked):

- roasted chickpeas

- spiced lentils

- lightly fried organic tofu or tempeh

- shredded, boiled organic, pasture-raised chicken or turkey

- hard-boiled organic, pasture-raised egg

Add your vegetables (at least 3):

- fresh leafy greens like spinach, arugula, or watercress

- crispy raw veggies like cucumber, bell peppers, shredded carrots, shredded red cabbage, radish, broccoli sprouts

- steamed veggies like organic edamame,

- roasted veggies like sweet potatoes, broccoli, cauliflower, carrots, Brussels sprouts, squash

Get creative with fresh herbs

- fresh cilantro, basil, parsley, dill, or chives add fresh bursts of flavor

Finalize with healthy fats:

- Fresh avocado

- Raw nuts and seeds

- Homemade dressings, like tahini, peanut sauce or pesto

Bonus: fermented foods

- naturally fermented foods like sauerkraut, kimchi, miso, or some pickled veggies are powerful probiotics, great for gut health and full of intense flavor

Directions

Cook your base and proteins ahead of time so that you have them ready to incorporate into a bowl in a moment's notice. If you're going to cook any vegetables, have those pre-cooked as well.

To prepare your meal, get a large bowl or glass Tupperware container if you're bringing it to go.

Start with your base, using 2/3 – 1 cup of cooked quinoa, lentils, beans, or rice per serving. Add a small portion, about the size of your fist, of your prepared additional proteins. Add plenty of vegetables and herbs as much as you can eat. Decorate with any fermented foods, nuts, or seeds you'd like to add.

Finally, add your dressing when you're ready to eat.

This is a filling meal, so you won't be hungry again quickly, but the fresh vegetables will provide you with steady energy, and the healthy fats will make sure your brain powers you through the rest of the day. If this is your lunch, you don't have to worry about the mid-afternoon slump.

Super Soup

Soups are an amazing way to pack a lot of nutrition into a single meal and, if you're dealing with picky eaters, you can easily hide a wide variety of vegetables simply by pureeing them before adding them to the soup.

Ingredients

Choose one or a combination for your soup base:

- bone broth

- vegetable broth

- water plus stewed and pureed tomatoes

Add extra flavor to any of these options by sautéing onions, garlic, and celery in a small about of olive oil and then adding to your base.

Choose your protein:

- organic, pasture-raised chicken or turkey

- wild or brown rice

- lentils, chickpeas or black beans

- quinoa

- organic tofu

You can also add nutritional yeast for a healthy burst of flavor that is also high in vitamins, minerals, and protein. It creates a nutty, slightly cheesy flavor.

Add your vegetables (at least 3):

- leafy greens like kale, chard, spinach, arugula, or beet greens

- cruciferous vegetables such as shredded cabbage, broccoli, cauliflower, bok choy, or Brussels sprouts

- root veggies like sweet potatoes, carrots, turnips, parsnips, beets, or fennel

- squashes, such as pumpkin, butternut, zucchini or summer squash

While you can leave squash in hearty, bite-sized cubes, pre-cooking and pureeing them make for a creamy, subtly sweet soup base.

Select fresh or dried herbs:

- rosemary, thyme, oregano, parsley and basil each play out very well in soup, but don't hesitate to experiment with your own favorites

Directions

The easiest way to make a big batch of soup is to use a slow cooker. Add all your ingredients in the morning before you go to work or get on with the business of your day and put it on low. A crockpot will be safe to leave on whether or not you're home, and will slowly simmer your soup to perfection over the next 6 – 8 hours.

If you don't have a slow cooker, you can add all your ingredients to a large stockpot and cook over medium to low heat for 1 – 3 hours, stirring occasionally.

You can cook soup quicker, if you are diligent in watching the stove and frequently stirring, allowing for a low boil.

Most soups freeze incredibly effectively, so making a large batch to save some for future quick meal solutions is a time and money-saving plan.

Stuffed Veggies

Many vegetables lend themselves very well to being stuffed. This is a great way to make a vitamin-packed vegetable the star of your meal, supported by the remaining ingredients. If you've become overly reliant on pasta and rice and you're struggling to make easy meals without these high-glycemic carbs, stuffed veggies are a creative alternative for dinner.

Ingredients

Vegetables that stuff well:

- bell peppers

- tomatoes

- acorn squash

- eggplant, zucchini or summer squash

- artichokes

- avocado

- portobello mushrooms

You can also use cabbage, collard greens, or other large green leaves to "wrap" your filling instead of getting stuffed.

Alternatively, baked potatoes and sweet potatoes can have their insides scooped out and mashed, added to the filling, and then stuffed.

Pick your protein (pre-cook):

- shredded, boiled organic, pasture-raised chicken or turkey

- crumbled organic tofu or tempeh

- lentils or black beans

- quinoa

- wild or brown rice

- organic edamame

Add your vegetables (at least 2):

- finely chopped fresh leafy greens like spinach, kale, arugula, beet greens or swiss chard

- finely cubed pieces of carrot, bell pepper, broccoli, cauliflower, and the edible centers of any vegetable you are planning on stuffing

- sautéed onion, garlic and/or celery for added flavor

Directions

Pre-cook your protein.

Clean and empty the center of the vegetable you have chosen to stuff. If you're using bell peppers, you can discard the seeds, but the centers of all the other options can be re-incorporated into the filling to avoid waste.

Combine your cooked protein and your vegetables together in a large bowl.

Fill your primary vegetables and roast in the oven for 20 – 40 minutes, depending on the vegetable you've chosen.

If you're stuffing a hearty squash, like acorn, you might want to pre-cook it halfway before stuffing it in order to avoid either undercooking the squash or overcooking the filling.

Spiced Chia Pudding

This incredibly easy to make dessert or meal replacement is high in protein, fiber, and, depending on your unique additions, flavor.

You can make it without sugar or dairy, making it a diabetic, gluten-free, vegan-friendly dessert that can be eaten in place of any meal without guilt.

Ingredients

The only two mandatory ingredients are:

- chia seeds

- milk or milk alternative

For the biggest health impact, choose organic, unsweetened options.

Depending on where you are in the reset and your own unique food sensitivities, you have a wide variety of added flavors that you can enhance your chia pudding with. The fruit is the most popular option, but it's not exclusive.

- Pureed fruit, such as pineapple, stewed apples, or berries

- Nut or seed butter

- Dark chocolate

- Fresh or dried coconut

Adding fresh or dried spices can also incorporate big flavor without the sugar-load pitfall. A few great combinations include:

- Cinnamon, nutmeg, cloves, allspice

- Ginger and turmeric, with a touch of cayenne

- Ginger and cinnamon

- Mint

Directions

To make your pudding, simply soak ¼ cup of chia seeds in 1 cup of milk or milk alternative for at least an hour, refrigerated.

When the chia has soaked up all the milk, you can add your pureed flavorings and spices. For a textured pudding, just mix in the additions, and for a smoother, more traditional pudding mouth feel, blend everything together.

Serve cooled.